HERBAL ALCHEMY:

UNLEASHING THE POTENCY OF NATURE'S ELIXIRS

By: Tanya Smith

TABLE OF CONTENTS

1. INTRODUCTION

2. GETTING STARTED WITH TINCTURE MAKING

3. KEY INGREDIENTS FOR TINCTURES

- Ginger: Digestive Aid

- Thyme: Respiratory Health

- Meadowsweet: Pain Relief

- Mullein: Respiratory Health

- Passion Flower: Sleep Aid

- St. John's Wort: Mood Support

- California Poppy: Relaxation

- Other Herbs and Their Uses

4. TINCTURE RECIPES AND PREPARATION METHODS

- Detailed instructions for each tincture, including herb ratios and extraction techniques

5. STORAGE AND DOSAGE GUIDELINES

- Proper storage methods to maintain potency
- Dosage guidelines for different ailments and populations

6. COMMON AILMENTS AND RECOMMENDED TINCTURE COMBINATIONS

- In-depth explanations of how each tincture can help specific ailments
- Suggested combinations for enhanced effectiveness

7. CONCLUSION

- Harnessing the Power of Nature for Wellness

In the fast-paced modern world, many of us are seeking natural alternatives to support our health and well-being. Enter the world of herbal tinctures—a hidden treasure trove of nature's miracles waiting to be discovered. Welcome to "Herbal Alchemy: Unleashing the Potency of Nature's Elixirs."

In this captivating journey, we will dive deep into the enchanting world of herbal tinctures, unlocking their secrets and unveiling their immense power. From ancient remedies passed down through generations to modern innovations, prepare to be awestruck by the myriad benefits these herbal elixirs can offer.

Throughout this book, you will embark on a quest to understand the science behind herbal tinctures and their remarkable healing properties. We will explore the art of crafting tinctures, uncovering the ancient wisdom of herbalists and their finely tuned methods. You will learn how each herb holds a unique key to unlocking the potential within your body and mind.

But the magic doesn't stop there. "Herbal Alchemy" will guide you through a journey of self-discovery, as you harness the power of nature to enhance your well-being. From boosting your immune system to reducing stress and promoting vitality, you will discover a world of natural remedies that can transform your life.

So, brace yourself for an immersive adventure into the world of "Herbal Alchemy: Unleashing the Potency of Nature's Elixirs." Are you ready to unlock the secrets of herbal tinctures and unleash their transformative power? Let the journey begin!

CHAPTER 1

Herbal tinctures are potent liquid extracts that have been used for centuries to reap the benefits of various medicinal plants. These extracts are made by steeping herbs in a solvent, typically alcohol or glycerin, which helps capture and preserve the plant's active compounds.

One of the key advantages of herbal tinctures is their ability to deliver the therapeutic properties of herbs in a concentrated and easily absorbable form. When taken orally, tinctures allow the body to quickly and efficiently absorb the beneficial compounds, making them ideal for addressing specific health concerns.

Herbal tinctures offer a wide range of benefits, including:

ENHANCED POTENCY:

Tinctures are highly concentrated, allowing for a higher concentration of active plant compounds compared to other preparations like teas or capsules.

LONGER SHELF LIFE:

The alcohol or glycerin base in tinctures acts as a natural preservative, prolonging the shelf life of the herbs and maintaining their efficacy.

CUSTOMIZABILITY:

Tinctures offer the flexibility to combine various herbs to create unique formulas tailored to specific health needs or preferences.

RAPID ABSORPTION:

Tinctures are quickly absorbed into the bloodstream, allowing for faster response times and more immediate effects.

CONVENIENT AND PORTABLE:

Tinctures are easy to carry and use on the go, making them a convenient option for busy lifestyles.

VERSATILITY:

Tinctures can be used internally by consuming them directly or adding them to drinks, or externally by applying them topically.

It is important to note that while herbal tinctures can provide numerous benefits, they should be used responsibly and under the guidance of a healthcare professional. Some individuals may have sensitivities or allergies to certain herbs, and proper dosage and administration are crucial for safe and effective use.

In this book, we will explore a variety of herbal tincture recipes, their health benefits, and proper usage guidelines. Whether you are new to herbalism or a seasoned practitioner, this book aims to provide valuable insights and inspiration to harness the power of herbal tinctures for your well-being.

UNDERSTANDING ALCOHOL-BASED EXTRACTION

Alcohol-based extraction is a commonly used method to obtain the beneficial compounds from various plant materials. This process involves soaking the plant material in alcohol, allowing it to macerate over time, and then filtering out the liquid to create an extract. This technique is widely used
in herbal medicine, perfumery, and the creation of various botanical products.

Alcohol-based extraction offers several advantages that make it a popular choice for obtaining plant extracts:

SOLUBILITY:

Alcohol has the ability to dissolve a wide range of plant compounds, including essential oils, alkaloids, and flavonoids. This makes it an effective solvent for extracting various beneficial components from plants.

PRESERVATION:

Alcohol acts as a natural preservative, helping to extend the shelf life of plant extracts by inhibiting microbial growth and oxidation. This ensures that the extract remains potent and effective over an extended period.

VERSATILITY:

Alcohol-based extraction can be used with a wide variety of plant materials, allowing for the extraction of different types of compounds from a diverse range of plants. This versatility makes it a valuable technique in botanical research and herbal medicine.

CONCENTRATION:

Alcohol-based extraction can produce highly concentrated extracts, allowing for efficient and effective delivery of the plant's therapeutic properties. This is particularly beneficial in situations where a small amount of extract is required to achieve the desired effect.

EASE OF USE:

The process of alcohol-based extraction is relatively straightforward and can be done using readily available tools and materials. It is a method that can be easily adopted by both professionals and enthusiasts alike.

SAFETY:

Alcohol used in extraction is generally safe for consumption and is well-tolerated by most individuals. However, it is important to consider any potential sensitivities or allergies, and to use high-quality alcohol that is fit for consumption.

Understanding the principles and techniques behind alcohol-based extraction can open up a world of possibilities for creating herbal remedies, natural health products, and botanical preparations. By harnessing the power of this extraction method, you can unlock the full potential of various plants and experience their healing and aromatic benefits.

In this section, we will dive deeper into the process of alcohol-based extraction, exploring the different techniques and considerations involved. By gaining a thorough understanding of this extraction method, you will be equipped with the knowledge to create high-quality plant extracts and explore the vast realm of botanical possibilities.

CHAPTER 2

Choosing quality herbs is essential when it comes to tincture making. The quality of herbs directly impacts the effectiveness and potency of the resulting tincture. When selecting herbs for tincture making, it is important to consider factors such as freshness, purity, and potency.

Freshness of herbs plays a vital role in tincture making. Fresh herbs are rich in essential oils and active compounds, which are responsible for the therapeutic properties of the tincture. By using fresh herbs, you can ensure that the tincture will be more potent and effective in delivering the desired benefits.

Purity of herbs is another crucial factor to consider. It is important to source herbs from reputable suppliers who follow good manufacturing practices and ensure that their products are free from contaminants or adulterants. Purity ensures that the tincture is safe for consumption and free from any undesirable substances that may have adverse effects on health.

The potency of herbs also matters when making tinctures. Different varieties and species of the same herb can vary in their potency and concentration of active compounds. Choosing herbs that are known for their strong medicinal properties can result in a more potent tincture.

Choosing quality herbs for tincture making is of utmost importance to ensure the effectiveness and safety of the final product. Freshness, purity, and potency are essential factors to consider when selecting herbs for tincture making. By being mindful of these factors, you can create high-quality tinctures that have optimal therapeutic value.

Sourcing and harvesting herbs are critical steps in the tincture-making process. The way herbs are sourced and harvested can greatly impact the quality and effectiveness of the tincture. It is important to understand the importance of these steps to ensure you are using high-quality herbs for your tincture making.

Proper sourcing of herbs involves selecting reputable suppliers or, ideally, growing your own herbs. When sourcing herbs, it is crucial to consider factors such as the quality of the soil, cultivation methods, and potential exposure to pesticides or other chemicals. By knowing the source of your herbs, you can ensure that they have been grown and handled in a way that maximizes their potency and purity.

Harvesting herbs at the right time is equally important. The timing of the harvest can significantly impact the herb's concentration of active compounds. Some herbs are best harvested when their flowers are in full bloom, while others are optimal when the leaves are at their peak. It is essential to research each herb's specific harvesting requirements to ensure that you are obtaining the most potent and beneficial parts of the plant.

Proper harvesting techniques, such as using sharp and clean tools, gentle handling, and promptly drying the herbs, can help preserve their potency and prevent spoilage. Harvesting in the right conditions, such as during the early morning when the herbs' essential oils are at their peak, can further enhance the quality of the herbs and, consequently, the tincture.

Sourcing and harvesting high-quality herbs are vital steps in tincture making. By sourcing herbs from reputable suppliers or growing your own and harvesting them at the right time, you can ensure that the herbs used in your tinctures are fresh, potent, and free from contaminants. These steps ultimately contribute to the overall quality and efficacy of your tinctures.

Having the right equipment and supplies is essential when it comes to making tinctures. The right tools can make the process smoother, more efficient, and help maintain the quality of the final product. Let's delve into the importance of essential equipment and supplies for making tinctures.

To begin with, a high-quality mortar and pestle are vital for grinding and crushing herbs. This allows you to release the active compounds and maximize their extraction during the tincture-making process. Similarly, having a reliable scale is crucial for accurately measuring the herbs and alcohol ratios, ensuring consistency and potency in your tinctures. Additionally, glass jars or bottles with tight-fitting lids are necessary for storing and aging tinctures properly, keeping them protected from light and air.

Filtration materials, such as cheesecloth or a fine-mesh strainer, come in handy during the decanting process, allowing you to separate the liquid tincture from the solid herbs. Filter paper can also be used for finer filtration, ensuring a clean and debris-free tincture. Moreover, amber or dark-colored glass bottles are preferred for storing tinctures, as they help protect the tincture from light, which can degrade the active compounds.

Most importantly, using high-quality alcohol, such as vodka or grain alcohol, is key to extracting and preserving the medicinal properties of the herbs effectively. The alcohol acts as a solvent, extracting the herbal compounds and preserving them for long-term storage. Ensuring the alcohol used is of high quality and has a high percentage of alcohol content (at least 40% or higher) is crucial for the tincture's effectiveness and shelf life.

In conclusion, having the right equipment and supplies is vital for making tinctures. From mortar and pestle for grinding herbs to glass bottles for storing the final product, each tool plays a crucial role in the tincture-making process. The right equipment and supplies not only make the process easier but also help maintain the quality and potency of the tinctures you create.

CHAPTER 3

<u>REISHI: IMMUNE SUPPORT</u>

Reishi, also known as Ganoderma lucidum, is a powerful medicinal mushroom that has long been revered for its immune-supporting properties. It has been used in traditional medicine for centuries to promote overall health and vitality. Let's explore the immune-supporting benefits of Reishi and how it can help boost the body's defenses.

One of the key components of Reishi is its polysaccharides, which have shown to have immunomodulating effects. These polysaccharides stimulate the activity of white blood cells, such as macrophages and natural killer cells, which play a crucial role in the immune response. By enhancing the activity of these immune cells, Reishi helps strengthen the body's defense against pathogens, viruses, and harmful bacteria.

Reishi is also rich in antioxidants, which help combat oxidative stress and reduce inflammation in the body. Chronic inflammation can weaken the immune system and make the body more susceptible to infections and diseases. The antioxidants found in Reishi help neutralize free radicals and reduce inflammation, thereby supporting the immune system's ability to function optimally.

Reishi is known to have adaptogenic properties, which means it helps the body adapt to stress and promotes balance. Chronic stress can suppress the immune system, making individuals more prone to illness. By reducing stress and promoting relaxation, Reishi supports the immune system's ability to function effectively and maintain overall health.

In addition to its immune-supporting properties, Reishi is also believed to have anti-cancer and anti-tumor effects. Some studies have shown that Reishi extracts can inhibit the growth of certain types of cancer cells and enhance the body's natural defense mechanisms against cancer. While more research is needed in this area, the potential anti-cancer properties of Reishi are promising.

Reishi is a potent mushroom that offers numerous immune-supporting benefits. From stimulating immune cell activity to reducing inflammation and combating stress, Reishi can help strengthen the body's defenses and promote overall health and vitality. Whether consumed in extract form or used in traditional herbal preparations, Reishi is a valuable ally for supporting and maintaining a healthy immune system.

LION'S MANE: COGNITIVE HEALTH

Lion's Mane is a medicinal mushroom that has gained significant attention for its potential benefits on cognitive health. Studies have suggested that Lion's Mane may have a positive impact on brain function and mental well-being. This mushroom is rich in compounds called hericenones and erinacines, which have been found to stimulate the production of nerve growth factor (NGF) in the brain. NGF is essential for the growth, maintenance, and repair of neurons, supporting overall brain health.

By promoting the production of NGF, Lion's Mane may enhance neuron function and communication, potentially improving cognitive abilities such as learning, memory, and focus. Research has shown that Lion's Mane may have neuroprotective effects, helping to safeguard against age-related cognitive decline and preventing the development of neurodegenerative diseases, such as Alzheimer's and Parkinson's.

Lion's Mane has also been associated with mood-enhancing properties. It may help reduce symptoms of anxiety and depression by modulating neurotransmitters in the brain, such as serotonin and dopamine. It is important to note that while Lion's Mane shows promising potential, further research is still needed to fully understand its mechanisms and benefits for cognitive health. Nonetheless, it is considered a safe and natural supplement that has gained popularity among individuals looking to support their brain health and overall cognitive function.

CORDYCEPS: ENERGY AND STAMINA

Cordyceps is a type of mushroom that has long been used in traditional Chinese medicine for its potential benefits on energy and stamina. It is believed to have adaptogenic properties, meaning it helps the body adapt and cope with physical and mental stress. Cordyceps is rich in bioactive compounds, such as cordycepin and adenosine, which have been found to improve energy production and oxygen utilization in the body.

One of the key benefits of Cordyceps is its ability to enhance athletic performance and boost overall physical endurance. Research suggests that Cordyceps may improve oxygen uptake by increasing the production of a compound called adenosine triphosphate (ATP) in the cells. ATP is the primary source of energy in the body, and by increasing its availability, Cordyceps may help athletes and individuals engaged in physical activities to perform at their best for longer periods.

In addition to its effects on physical energy and stamina, Cordyceps may also have positive impacts on mental well-being and cognitive function. It is believed to improve blood flow to the brain and support the production of neurotransmitters that are essential for optimal brain health. By reducing fatigue and enhancing mental clarity, Cordyceps may help individuals maintain focus and concentration throughout the day.

While more research is needed to fully understand the mechanisms and benefits of Cordyceps, it has gained popularity as a natural supplement to support energy, stamina, and overall physical performance. It is important to consult with a healthcare professional before starting any new supplement regimen, especially if you have any underlying health conditions or are taking medications.

TURKEY TAIL: GUT HEALTH

Turkey Tail, scientifically known as Trametes versicolor, is a type of mushroom that has been used for centuries in traditional medicine, particularly in Asian countries. Among its many potential benefits, Turkey Tail is known for its positive effects on gut health. It contains an abundance of polysaccharides, including beta-glucans, which have been found to support a healthy gut microbiome.

The gut microbiome refers to the trillions of microorganisms that reside in our digestive system. Maintaining a healthy balance of these microorganisms is crucial for overall health and well-being. Research has shown that Turkey Tail can help promote the growth of beneficial bacteria in the gut, such as Bifidobacterium and Lactobacillus, while inhibiting the growth of harmful bacteria. This supports a balanced gut microbiome, which is essential for proper digestion, nutrient absorption, immune function, and even mental health.

Turkey Tail is rich in prebiotics, which are fibers that serve as food for the beneficial bacteria in our gut. By providing nourishment to these bacteria, Turkey Tail helps them thrive and perform their important roles. A healthy gut microbiome has been linked to improved digestion, reduced risk of gastrointestinal disorders, enhanced immune function, and even a positive impact on conditions like irritable bowel syndrome (IBS) and inflammatory bowel disease (IBD).

While more research is needed to fully understand the potential benefits of Turkey Tail for gut health, its long history of use in traditional medicine and promising preliminary studies suggest that it can be a valuable natural supplement to support a healthy digestive system. As always, it is recommended to consult with a healthcare professional before starting any new supplement regimen, especially if you have any underlying health conditions or are taking medications.

NETTLE: ALLERGY RELIEF

Nettle, scientifically known as Urtica dioica, is a perennial plant that has been used for centuries as herbal medicine. Among its many potential benefits, Nettle is particularly known for its ability to provide relief from allergies. It is a natural antihistamine and anti-inflammatory herb that can help alleviate symptoms associated with seasonal allergies like sneezing, itching, nasal congestion, and watery eyes.

When we come into contact with allergens such as pollen, our immune system releases histamines, which trigger an allergic response. Nettle contains several bioactive compounds, including histamine inhibitors, that can help counteract the effects of histamine release in the body. By inhibiting the production of histamine, Nettle can help reduce the severity of allergy symptoms.

Nettle has anti-inflammatory properties that can help soothe inflammation in the respiratory system. Allergies often cause inflammation in the nasal passages and airways, leading to congestion and difficulty in breathing. The anti-inflammatory compounds found in Nettle can help alleviate these symptoms and promote clear breathing.

Studies have shown that Nettle extract can be effective in relieving symptoms of allergic rhinitis, which is a common type of seasonal allergy. It is generally well-tolerated and can be used as an alternative to over-the-counter antihistamine medications. However, it is important to note that the effectiveness of Nettle may vary among individuals, and it is recommended to consult with a healthcare professional before incorporating it into your allergy management plan.

Nettle is a natural remedy that offers potential relief from allergies. Its antihistamine and anti-inflammatory properties make it a valuable herb for alleviating symptoms associated with seasonal allergies. If you are seeking a natural approach to managing your allergies, Nettle may be worth considering, but as always, it is advisable to consult with a healthcare professional for personalized advice and guidance.

ECHINACEA: COLD AND FLU DEFENSE

Echinacea, also known as purple coneflower, is a flowering plant that has been used for centuries as a traditional remedy for boosting the immune system and fighting off colds and the flu. It is known for its potent medicinal properties and is particularly recognized for its ability to enhance the body's natural defense mechanisms.

One of the key benefits of Echinacea is its immune-stimulating properties. It contains a variety of active compounds, such as flavonoids and polysaccharides, which can help enhance the activity of immune cells and strengthen the body's immune response. By supporting and boosting the immune system, Echinacea can potentially help defend against common cold and flu viruses.

In addition to its immune-boosting properties, Echinacea also exhibits antiviral and antibacterial effects. Research has found that certain compounds in Echinacea can inhibit the growth and replication of viruses and bacteria, which are often responsible for causing respiratory infections. This makes Echinacea a valuable natural remedy not only for colds and the flu but also for other respiratory infections.

While Echinacea is generally considered safe, it is important to note that its effectiveness may vary among individuals. It is recommended to take it at the earliest sign of symptoms and to follow the recommended dosage guidelines. As with any supplement or herbal remedy, it's always a good idea to consult with a healthcare professional, especially if you have any underlying health conditions or concerns.

Echinacea is a natural remedy that has gained popularity for its potential immune-boosting and anti-viral properties. By supporting the immune system and providing antiviral effects, Echinacea can play a role in defending against colds and the flu. However, it's important to remember that individual results may vary, and it's always best to seek guidance from a healthcare professional for personalized advice and recommendations.

LICORICE ROOT: RESPIRATORY SUPPORT

Licorice root is a powerful herb widely used for its numerous health benefits, including its ability to provide respiratory support. With a history dating back centuries, licorice root has been traditionally used in Eastern and Western herbal medicine to address respiratory conditions such as coughs, asthma, and congestion.

Licorice root contains a compound called glycyrrhizin, which has been found to have expectorant properties. This means that it can help promote the removal of mucus and secretions from the respiratory tract, which makes it beneficial for those dealing with respiratory congestion or bronchitis. Licorice root is also known to soothe irritated tissues, which can provide relief for coughs and sore throats.

Another valuable component of licorice root is a substance called flavonoids. Flavonoids possess anti-inflammatory properties that can help reduce inflammation in the respiratory system. By reducing inflammation, licorice root can help ease symptoms of respiratory conditions and promote better breathing.

Licorice root has been found to have antiviral and antimicrobial properties. This means that it may have the ability to inhibit the growth of certain respiratory viruses and bacteria, providing a potential line of defense against respiratory infections.

It is important to note that while licorice root offers potential respiratory support, it should be used in moderation and under the guidance of a healthcare professional. Prolonged or excessive use of licorice root can have adverse effects, such as increasing blood pressure or impairing kidney function. Pregnant women, individuals with high blood pressure, and those with certain medical conditions should exercise caution and consult with a healthcare provider before using licorice root.

Licorice root can be a valuable herb for respiratory support. Its expectorant and anti-inflammatory properties can help alleviate congestion, coughs, and sore throats. Additionally, its antiviral and antimicrobial properties provide potential protection against respiratory infections. However, it's important to use licorice root responsibly and seek professional guidance to ensure safe and effective use.

RASPBERRY LEAF: WOMEN'S HEALTH

Raspberry leaf is an herb that has long been valued for its medicinal uses, particularly in supporting women's health. The leaves of the raspberry plant (Rubus idaeus) contain a variety of beneficial compounds that have been traditionally used to address menstrual discomfort, promote healthy pregnancy and childbirth, and support overall reproductive health.

One of the key benefits of raspberry leaf is its ability to alleviate menstrual cramps and discomfort. It is believed that the high concentration of fragrine, an alkaloid found in raspberry leaves, helps to tone and strengthen the muscles of the uterus, reducing the intensity of menstrual cramps. By relaxing the uterine muscles, raspberry leaf can also help regulate menstrual cycles and promote a more balanced hormonal environment.

Raspberry leaf has been praised for its potential benefits during pregnancy. Many women choose to consume raspberry leaf tea or take raspberry leaf supplements during their third trimester to prepare for labor and childbirth. It is believed that raspberry leaf can help tone and strengthen the uterine muscles, which may enhance the efficiency of contractions and shorten labor duration. Some studies have suggested that women who consume raspberry leaf during pregnancy may experience a reduced need for interventions such as artificial rupture of membranes or cesarean section.

Furthermore, raspberry leaf is considered a rich source of vitamins and minerals that can support overall reproductive health. It contains essential nutrients like calcium, iron, magnesium, and B vitamins, which are important for menstrual regularity, fertility, and overall wellbeing. Raspberry leaf also has antioxidant properties that may help protect against cellular damage and promote a healthy reproductive system.

It is important to note that while raspberry leaf is generally considered safe for most women to use, it is recommended to consult with a healthcare professional before incorporating it into your routine, especially during pregnancy. They can provide personalized advice on dosage and any potential interactions or contraindications based on your specific health needs.

Raspberry leaf is a herb known for its beneficial effects on women's health. Its ability to alleviate menstrual discomfort, support a healthy pregnancy, and provide essential nutrients make it a popular choice for many women. However, it is crucial to seek professional guidance to ensure safe and appropriate use, particularly during pregnancy.

ELDERBERRIES: IMMUNE BOOSTER

Elderberries are small, dark purple berries that come from the elder tree, scientifically known as Sambucus nigra. These berries have long been celebrated for their potential immune-boosting properties and have been used in traditional remedies for centuries. The immune-boosting effects of elderberries can be attributed to their high content of antioxidants, particularly anthocyanins, which give the berries their deep purple color.

Research suggests that elderberries may help enhance the immune system's response to common colds and flu. The antioxidants in elderberries can help reduce inflammation and oxidative stress in the body, which are associated with weakened immune function. Additionally, elderberries have been found to inhibit the replication of viruses, potentially shortening the duration and severity of respiratory infections.

The immune-boosting benefits of elderberries extend beyond fighting off colds and flu. Some studies suggest that elderberry extracts may also have antiviral properties against other viral strains, including those associated with herpes and certain strains of influenza. Moreover, elderberries have been found to stimulate the production of certain immune cells, such as cytokines, which play a crucial role in the body's defense against pathogens.

Besides their immune-boosting effects, elderberries are also rich in vitamins, such as vitamin C and vitamin A, as well as other beneficial nutrients like fiber and flavonoids. These nutrients contribute to the overall health of the body and can support general wellbeing.

It is worth noting that while elderberries are generally considered safe, it is important to use them in moderation and in appropriate forms. Consuming raw or unripe elderberries can be toxic, so it is best to use commercially prepared products, such as elderberry syrups or supplements, that have been properly processed to remove any potential toxins.

Elderberries are a powerful immune booster due to their high antioxidant content and potential antiviral properties. Incorporating elderberries into your diet or using elderberry-based products may help support your immune system, reduce the duration of respiratory infections, and promote overall wellbeing. However, always ensure you are using properly prepared elderberry products and consult a healthcare professional if you have any concerns or underlying medical conditions.

ASHWAGANDHA: STRESS RELIEF

Ashwagandha, also known as Withania somnifera or Indian ginseng, is an ancient medicinal herb that has been used for centuries in Ayurvedic medicine. It is renowned for its adaptogenic properties, which means it helps the body adapt to stress and promotes overall balance and well-being. Stress has become a common issue in our modern lives, and finding effective ways to manage it is crucial for our physical and mental health.

One of the key benefits of ashwagandha is its ability to help regulate the body's stress response. It works by reducing the levels of cortisol, often referred to as the "stress hormone," which can have a negative impact on various aspects of health when chronically elevated. By lowering cortisol levels, ashwagandha can help alleviate symptoms of stress, such as anxiety, irritability, and fatigue.

In addition to its stress-reducing effects, ashwagandha has been shown to have numerous other health benefits. It has been traditionally used to enhance cognitive function and improve memory. Research suggests that ashwagandha may help promote healthy brain function by reducing oxidative stress, supporting the growth of nerve cells, and regulating neurotransmitters involved in memory and learning.

Ashwagandha also has potential immune-supporting properties. Chronic stress can weaken the immune system, making individuals more susceptible to infections and illnesses. Ashwagandha's adaptogenic effects may help strengthen immune function by regulating immune responses and reducing inflammation in the body.

Furthermore, ashwagandha has been found to have mood-stabilizing properties, potentially aiding in the management of conditions like depression and anxiety. It may enhance the activity of neurotransmitters such as serotonin and GABA, which play a crucial role in regulating mood and emotions.

It is important to note that while ashwagandha is generally considered safe for most individuals, it may interact with certain medications or have side effects in some cases. It is always best to consult with a healthcare professional before starting any new supplement, especially if you have underlying health conditions or are taking medications.

Ashwagandha is a valuable herb known for its stress-relieving and adaptogenic properties. By helping to regulate stress hormone levels, supporting cognitive function, boosting immune health, and potentially improving mood, ashwagandha can be a beneficial addition to promote overall well-being. However, it is essential to consult with a healthcare provider for personalized advice and guidance on proper dosage and usage.

MARSHMALLOW ROOT: DIGESTIVE SOOTHER

Marshmallow root, also known as Althaea officinalis, is an herb that has a long history of use in traditional medicine, particularly for its soothing effects on the digestive system. It has been used for centuries to relieve various digestive issues, such as acid reflux, gastritis, and irritable bowel syndrome.

One of the key benefits of marshmallow root is its mucilaginous properties. It contains a high concentration of mucilage, a thick, gel-like substance that forms a protective coating on the lining of the digestive tract. This coating helps to soothe and protect the mucous membranes, reducing inflammation and irritation. Additionally, marshmallow root can help to lubricate the intestines, softening the stool and easing constipation.

Marshmallow root is also known for its demulcent properties, which means it can help to relax and soften tissues. This can be particularly beneficial for individuals with conditions like gastritis or ulcers, as it can help to soothe the inflamed and irritated tissues in the stomach and intestines.

Moreover, marshmallow root has been used to help alleviate symptoms of acid reflux. It can help to neutralize excess stomach acid, reducing the discomfort and burning sensation associated with acid reflux. Marshmallow root can also help to improve overall digestion by promoting the healthy balance of gut bacteria.

It's important to note that while marshmallow root is generally considered safe for most individuals, it may interact with certain medications or have side effects in some cases. It is always best to consult with a healthcare professional before starting any new supplement, especially if you have underlying health conditions or are taking medications.

Marshmallow root is a valuable herb known for its soothing and protective effects on the digestive system. By providing relief from inflammation, irritation, and digestive discomfort, marshmallow root can be a helpful natural remedy for individuals with various digestive issues. However, it's important to seek guidance from a healthcare provider for personalized advice and recommendations on proper dosage and usage.

ROSEMARY: MENTAL CLARITY

Rosemary (Rosmarinus officinalis) is an aromatic herb that has been treasured for its culinary and medicinal uses for centuries. While it is widely known for its delightful flavor and fragrance, Rosemary also possesses several properties that can promote mental clarity and cognitive function.

One of the key components of Rosemary is rosmarinic acid, which has been found to have neuroprotective effects. Studies have suggested that rosmarinic acid can help to protect the brain against oxidative stress and inflammation, which are known to contribute to cognitive decline and memory impairment. By reducing oxidative damage and inflammation, Rosemary may support brain health and potentially improve memory and concentration.

The scent of Rosemary has been associated with enhanced cognitive performance. Research has shown that the aroma of Rosemary can have a positive impact on memory and alertness. In one study, exposure to the scent of Rosemary was found to improve prospective memory, which refers to the ability to remember to perform tasks in the future.

Rosemary also contains compounds that may have a positive influence on mood and stress levels. For example, Rosemary contains an essential oil called 1,8-cineole, which has been shown to have anxiolytic (anti-anxiety) and antidepressant effects. By reducing anxiety and promoting a more positive mood, Rosemary may help to enhance mental clarity and focus.

Incorporating Rosemary into your daily routine can be as simple as adding it to your meals, using it in herbal teas, or enjoying its aroma through essential oils or dried bouquets. However, it's important to note that Rosemary should not be used excessively or by individuals with certain health conditions or medications. As always, it's a good idea to consult with a healthcare professional before incorporating any new herbs or supplements into your routine.

In conclusion, Rosemary is not only a flavorful herb but also a beneficial ally for mental clarity. Its neuroprotective, memory-enhancing, and mood-boosting properties make it a valuable addition to a healthy lifestyle. So, next time you're seeking mental clarity, consider incorporating Rosemary in your daily routine and experience the potential cognitive benefits it has to offer.

<u>CHAMOMILE: CALMING ANXIETY</u>

Chamomile is a gentle and soothing herb that has been used for centuries for its calming and anxiety-reducing properties. It is widely known for its ability to promote relaxation, relieve stress, and improve sleep quality.

One of the main compounds in Chamomile responsible for its calming effects is apigenin, a flavonoid with sedative and anxiolytic properties. Apigenin binds to specific receptors in the brain that help to reduce anxiety and promote feelings of calmness. This makes Chamomile a natural and safe alternative for managing anxiety symptoms.

Research has shown that Chamomile can be especially beneficial for individuals with generalized anxiety disorder (GAD). In a study conducted on individuals with GAD, Chamomile extract was found to significantly reduce symptoms of anxiety compared to a placebo group. The participants reported feeling more relaxed and had improved overall well-being.

Chamomile's effects on sleep can also contribute to its ability to calm anxiety. By promoting restful sleep, Chamomile helps to reduce fatigue and irritability, factors that can worsen anxiety symptoms. It has been found to have mild sedative effects, which can aid in falling asleep faster and having a more restorative sleep.

Incorporating Chamomile into your daily routine can be as simple as brewing a cup of Chamomile tea, taking a Chamomile supplement, or using Chamomile essential oil for aromatherapy. It is important to note that while Chamomile is generally safe for most people, some individuals may experience allergies or interactions with certain medications. As always, it is best to consult with a healthcare professional before introducing any new herbs or supplements into your routine, especially if you have pre-existing health conditions or are taking medications.

Chamomile is a natural remedy that can provide relief from anxiety and promote a sense of calmness. Its ability to reduce anxiety symptoms, improve sleep quality, and induce relaxation makes it a valuable tool for managing stress and anxiety. So, the next time you find yourself feeling anxious or overwhelmed, consider reaching for a cup of Chamomile tea and experience the soothing benefits it has to offer.

<u>ROSE: SKIN HEALTH</u>

Rose is known for more than just its beautiful appearance and pleasant fragrance—it also offers a wide range of benefits for skin health. Thanks to its high content of vitamins, antioxidants, and essential fatty acids, rose can be a valuable addition to any skincare routine.

One of the key benefits of rose for skin health is its moisturizing properties. Its natural oils help to lock in moisture and prevent water loss, keeping the skin hydrated and supple. This is particularly beneficial for individuals with dry or dehydrated skin, as it can help to alleviate dryness and restore a healthy moisture balance.

Rose is also rich in antioxidants, which can help to protect the skin from environmental damage and premature aging caused by free radicals. These harmful molecules contribute to the breakdown of collagen and elastin, resulting in wrinkles, fine lines, and sagging skin. The antioxidants found in rose help to neutralize free radicals, promoting a more youthful and radiant complexion.

In addition to its moisturizing and antioxidant properties, rose has anti-inflammatory effects that can soothe and calm irritated skin. It can help to reduce redness, inflammation, and other skin conditions such as rosacea and eczema. The natural healing properties of rose can also aid in the repair of damaged skin, helping to improve overall skin texture and tone.

Rose has a natural astringent effect, which can help to tighten and tone the skin. This can be particularly beneficial for individuals with oily or acne-prone skin, as it can help to reduce excess oil production and minimize the appearance of pores. It can also aid in the healing of acne scars and blemishes, promoting a clearer and smoother complexion.

Rose can be incorporated into your skincare routine in various forms, such as rose water, rosehip oil, or rose essential oil. Whether you choose to use it as a toner, moisturizer, or in a face mask, incorporating rose into your skincare routine can provide numerous benefits for your skin health.

In conclusion, rose is a versatile and beneficial ingredient for skin health. Its moisturizing, antioxidant, anti-inflammatory, and astringent properties make it a valuable addition to any skincare routine. By incorporating rose-based products into your regimen, you can nourish and protect your skin, promote a youthful complexion, and enhance overall skin health.

<u>DANDELION: LIVER SUPPORT</u>

Dandelion, often regarded as an invasive weed, actually offers numerous health benefits, particularly when it comes to supporting liver health. The liver plays a crucial role in detoxification, filtering out toxins and waste products from the bloodstream. Dandelion has long been used as a natural remedy to support liver function and promote overall liver health.

One of the key benefits of dandelion for liver support is its potent antioxidant properties. The plant is rich in antioxidants, such as beta-carotene, vitamin C, and polyphenols, which help to protect the liver cells from oxidative damage caused by free radicals. This protection is essential as the liver is constantly exposed to toxins from our environment, diet, and medications.

Another notable aspect of dandelion is its ability to stimulate liver function and promote the production of digestive enzymes. This can help to enhance the liver's ability to metabolize and eliminate toxins, helping to improve overall liver function and detoxification capabilities. Dandelion can also support healthy bile production, aiding in the breakdown and digestion of fats.

Furthermore, dandelion possesses diuretic properties, meaning it helps to increase urine production. This can be beneficial for the liver as it helps to flush out toxins and excess water from the body. By promoting optimal kidney function, dandelion indirectly supports the liver's detoxification process, reducing the burden on the liver itself.

Incorporating dandelion into your diet is relatively easy. The greens can be enjoyed in salads or cooked like other leafy greens, providing a rich source of vitamins, minerals, and antioxidants. Dandelion root can be consumed as a tea or taken in supplement form to promote liver health.

Dandelion is a powerful herb that offers significant benefits for liver support. Its antioxidant properties, ability to enhance liver function, and diuretic effects make it valuable in promoting liver health and detoxification. Adding dandelion to your diet or utilizing dandelion supplements can be a natural and effective way to support your liver and overall well-being.

BURDOCK: BLOOD PURIFICATION

Burdock, a root vegetable often overlooked, provides numerous health benefits, especially when it comes to blood purification. The process of blood purification is essential for maintaining overall health as it helps to remove toxins, waste products, and impurities from the bloodstream. Burdock has long been used in traditional medicine as a natural remedy to support blood purification and promote optimal health.

One of the key reasons why burdock is beneficial for blood purification is its powerful detoxifying properties. The root contains active compounds, such as inulin and phenolic acids, which have been shown to help eliminate toxins from the body. These compounds work by stimulating the kidneys and promoting increased urine production, helping to flush out waste products from the bloodstream.

Additionally, burdock is known for its blood-cleansing abilities. It contains compounds called lignans which have been found to have antimicrobial properties, helping to inhibit the growth of bacteria and fungi. This can be particularly beneficial in supporting the overall health of the blood and preventing infections.

Burdock is rich in antioxidants, such as quercetin and luteolin, which help to neutralize free radicals and reduce oxidative stress in the body. By reducing oxidative stress, burdock supports the health of the blood vessels and reduces inflammation, promoting a healthy circulatory system.

Incorporating burdock into your diet can be done in various ways. The root can be consumed raw, cooked, or juiced to enjoy its health benefits. It can be added to soups, stews, stir-fries, or even brewed as a tea. Burdock supplements are also available for those who prefer a more convenient option.

Burdock is a valuable root vegetable that offers significant benefits for blood purification. Its detoxifying properties, blood-cleansing abilities, and antioxidant content make it a valuable addition to a healthy lifestyle. Including burdock in your diet or utilizing burdock supplements can be a natural and effective way to support blood purification and promote optimal health.

<u>GINGER: DIGESTIVE AID</u>

Ginger is not only a popular spice in culinary applications but also a powerful digestive aid. For centuries, ginger has been used in traditional medicine to alleviate various digestive issues and promote healthy digestion. From relieving nausea to reducing bloating and indigestion, ginger offers a range of benefits for maintaining digestive health.

One of the key reasons why ginger is highly regarded as a digestive aid is its ability to reduce nausea and vomiting. Numerous studies have shown that ginger can effectively alleviate symptoms of motion sickness, morning sickness during pregnancy, and chemotherapy-induced nausea. It works by blocking certain receptors in the brain that trigger nausea, offering natural relief without any significant side effects.

In addition to its anti-nausea properties, ginger has been found to stimulate the digestive system and promote efficient digestion. It helps to increase the production of digestive enzymes, such as lipase and amylase, which aid in breaking down carbohydrates and fats, respectively. By enhancing the digestive process, ginger can aid in preventing common digestive complaints like bloating, indigestion, and flatulence.

Moreover, ginger possesses anti-inflammatory properties that can soothe the digestive system and alleviate inflammation in the gut. Chronic inflammation in the gastrointestinal tract can lead to symptoms like abdominal pain, diarrhea, and inflammatory bowel disease. The active compounds in ginger, such as gingerols and shogaols, help to reduce inflammation, providing relief from these symptoms and maintaining a healthy digestive system.

Including ginger in your diet is relatively easy. It can be consumed fresh, dried, powdered, or as a tea. Adding ginger to your meals, such as stir-fries, smoothies, or marinades, can help enhance digestion and provide a flavorful kick. Ginger tea can be enjoyed on its own or with added lemon and honey for a soothing and revitalizing beverage.

Ginger is a remarkable digestive aid with its anti-nausea properties, ability to stimulate digestion, and anti-inflammatory effects. Whether you're dealing with occasional digestive discomfort or seeking to maintain optimal digestive health, incorporating ginger into your daily routine can be a natural and effective way to support your digestive system.

THYME: RESPIRATORY HEALTH

Thyme is an herb that is not only known for its aromatic and culinary uses but also for its numerous health benefits, particularly in supporting respiratory health. For centuries, thyme has been used in traditional medicine to help alleviate respiratory conditions and promote overall lung health.

One of the key reasons why thyme is highly regarded for respiratory health is its expectorant properties. Thyme contains compounds such as thymol, which help to loosen and expel mucus from the airways. This makes it beneficial for individuals suffering from respiratory conditions such as bronchitis, coughs, and congestion. By promoting the elimination of mucus, thyme can help to clear the airways and ease breathing.

Thyme has been found to possess antimicrobial properties, making it effective against respiratory infections. Its active compounds have been shown to inhibit the growth of bacteria and fungi, including those that commonly cause respiratory infections like pneumonia and bronchitis. By fighting off these pathogens, thyme can help reduce the severity and duration of respiratory infections.

Thyme is rich in antioxidants, which help to protect the respiratory system from oxidative stress and damage caused by free radicals. Free radicals can contribute to the development of respiratory conditions and worsen symptoms. The antioxidants in thyme help to neutralize these harmful molecules, supporting the overall health and function of the respiratory system.

There are several ways to incorporate thyme into your routine to support respiratory health. It can be used in cooking to add flavor to dishes like soups, stews, and roasted vegetables. Thyme can also be used to make herbal teas or added to hot water for steam inhalation, providing a soothing and aromatic way to clear the airways.

Thyme is a valuable herb for maintaining respiratory health. Its expectorant, antimicrobial, and antioxidant properties make it a beneficial addition to any respiratory support regimen. Whether you prefer to use it in your cooking or as a herbal remedy, thyme offers a natural and effective way to promote healthy lungs and support optimal respiratory function.

MEADOWSWEET: PAIN RELIEF

Meadowsweet, also known as Filipendula ulmaria, is a natural herb that has long been valued for its pain-relieving properties. This perennial plant contains salicylates, the precursor to aspirin, which gives it its analgesic and anti-inflammatory effects. Meadowsweet has a rich history of use in traditional medicine for alleviating pain and discomfort associated with various conditions.

One of the primary benefits of using meadowsweet for pain relief is its ability to reduce inflammation. The salicylates present in meadowsweet help to inhibit the production of pro-inflammatory substances in the body, which can contribute to pain and swelling. By reducing inflammation, meadowsweet can provide relief from conditions such as arthritis, muscle aches, headaches, and menstrual cramps.

Meadowsweet has been found to have mild analgesic properties, meaning it can directly alleviate pain sensations. Its natural compounds work by blocking pain receptors in the body, providing a gentle and soothing effect. This makes meadowsweet a great option for individuals who prefer natural remedies for managing pain without relying solely on conventional medications.

Meadowsweet has a calming and relaxing effect on the body, which can help to ease tension and promote a sense of well-being. This can be particularly beneficial for individuals experiencing stress or anxiety-related pain. By calming the mind and body, meadowsweet can indirectly alleviate pain associated with these conditions.

There are several ways to enjoy the benefits of meadowsweet for pain relief. It can be brewed into a tea by steeping the dried or fresh flowers and leaves in hot water. The tea can be consumed up to three times a day to help manage pain and inflammation. Meadowsweet extracts and tinctures are also available and can be added to water or other beverages for ease of consumption.

Meadowsweet is a natural herb that offers effective pain relief without the potential side effects associated with conventional pain medications. Its anti-inflammatory and analgesic properties make it a valuable option for managing various types of pain, from arthritis to headaches. Whether enjoyed as a tea or taken in extract form, meadowsweet provides a natural and gentle approach to pain relief.

MULLEIN: RESPIRATORY HEALTH

Mullein, also known as Verbascum thapsus, is a flowering plant that has long been recognized for its numerous benefits for respiratory health. This herb has a rich history of use in traditional medicine, particularly as a remedy for various respiratory conditions. Mullein offers a range of therapeutic properties that promote healthy lungs and respiratory function.

One of the key benefits of mullein is its ability to soothe and calm respiratory inflammation. Its leaves contain mucilage, a gelatinous substance that has a soothing effect on irritated tissues. When consumed as a tea or inhaled as steam, mullein can help alleviate discomfort associated with conditions such as bronchitis, asthma, and coughs. The anti-inflammatory properties of mullein can also help reduce the production of excess mucus, making it easier to breathe.

Mullein possesses expectorant properties, which means it promotes the loosening and removal of mucus from the respiratory tract. This can be particularly beneficial for individuals with chest congestion or excessive phlegm. Mullein's expectorant effects help to clear the airways and facilitate easier breathing. As a natural remedy, mullein can be used as an herbal tea, tincture, or even inhaled through steam to help promote expectoration and relieve respiratory congestion.

Moreover, mullein has been found to have antimicrobial properties, which can help combat respiratory infections. It contains bioactive compounds that possess antibacterial and antiviral effects. These properties make mullein a valuable herb for supporting the immune system in fighting off respiratory infections and reducing their severity. By maintaining respiratory health and supporting the body's defenses, mullein can help protect against common respiratory ailments.

Mullein is an herb with significant benefits for respiratory health. Its ability to soothe inflammation, promote expectoration, and provide antimicrobial support make it a valuable natural remedy for managing respiratory conditions. Whether consumed as a tea or used in other forms, mullein offers a gentle and effective approach to supporting lung health and improving respiratory function.

PASSION FLOWER: SLEEP AID

Passion Flower, also known as Passiflora incarnata, is an herb that has been traditionally used for its calming and sedative effects. This beautiful flowering plant has gained popularity as a natural sleep aid due to its ability to promote relaxation and improve sleep quality.

One of the key benefits of Passion Flower is its ability to reduce anxiety and induce a state of calmness. It contains compounds that interact with the GABA receptors in the brain, which are responsible for regulating anxiety levels. By increasing the activity of GABA, Passion Flower helps to reduce feelings of restlessness and promotes a sense of tranquility. This can be particularly helpful for individuals who struggle with racing thoughts or have difficulty falling asleep due to anxiety.

Passion Flower has been found to have sedative properties, making it an excellent sleep aid. It can help lengthen the duration of sleep and improve the overall quality of sleep. By calming the mind and relaxing the body, Passion Flower can provide a natural solution for those experiencing insomnia or sleep disturbances. Its gentle sedative effects make it suitable for individuals who prefer a non-pharmaceutical approach to sleep aid.

In addition to its sleep-enhancing benefits, Passion Flower is also known for its overall relaxation and mood-improving effects. It can help reduce muscle tension, alleviate mild pain, and promote a sense of well-being. By promoting a state of relaxation, Passion Flower can also be beneficial for individuals experiencing stress-related sleep issues.

Passion Flower offers a natural and gentle solution for those seeking a sleep aid. Its ability to reduce anxiety, induce calmness, and promote sedation makes it a valuable herb for improving sleep quality. By incorporating Passion Flower into your sleep routine, you may experience a more restful and rejuvenating night's sleep.

ST. JOHN'S WORT: MOOD SUPPORT

St. John's Wort, scientifically known as Hypericum perforatum, is a herb that has long been used for its mood-enhancing properties. This flowering plant has gained significant attention as a natural remedy for supporting emotional well-being and relieving symptoms of mild depression and anxiety.

One of the key benefits of St. John's Wort is its ability to increase the levels of certain neurotransmitters in the brain, such as serotonin, dopamine, and noradrenaline. These neurotransmitters play a crucial role in regulating mood and emotions. By enhancing their availability, St. John's Wort can help alleviate feelings of sadness, improve overall mood, and promote a sense of well-being.

Research has shown that St. John's Wort may be effective in the treatment of mild to moderate depression. It has been found to be as effective as some conventional antidepressant medications, but with fewer side effects. However, it's important to note that St. John's Wort may interact with certain medications, so it is always advisable to consult with a healthcare professional before incorporating it into your routine.

In addition to its mood-enhancing properties, St. John's Wort also possesses anxiolytic effects, which means it may help reduce symptoms of anxiety. It has been reported to have a calming effect on the nervous system, promoting relaxation and reducing feelings of restlessness or nervousness. This makes it a valuable herb for individuals experiencing mild anxiety or stress-related mood disturbances.

St. John's Wort offers a natural alternative for supporting emotional well-being and promoting a positive mood. Its ability to increase neurotransmitter levels in the brain may help alleviate symptoms of mild depression and anxiety. However, it is important to consult with a healthcare professional before using St. John's Wort, especially if you are taking other medications, to ensure its safe and appropriate use.

CALIFORNIA POPPY: RELAXATION

California Poppy, scientifically known as Eschscholzia californica, is a flowering plant native to North America. It is widely recognized for its relaxing properties and has been traditionally used as a natural remedy for promoting calmness and alleviating stress and tension.

One of the key benefits of California Poppy is its ability to act as a mild sedative. Its compounds help soothe the nervous system and induce a state of relaxation, making it a popular choice for individuals looking to unwind after a long day or improve their sleep quality. California Poppy can help ease restlessness, irritability, and nervousness, allowing individuals to experience a sense of tranquility.

Furthermore, California Poppy is also known for its analgesic properties, which means it may help alleviate minor aches and pains. It has been used to treat headaches, muscle tension, and discomfort associated with nervous conditions. By promoting relaxation and reducing tension in the body, California Poppy can contribute to a greater sense of well-being and physical comfort.

California Poppy is typically consumed as a liquid extract or tea, and it is generally well-tolerated with few side effects. However, it is advised to consult with a healthcare professional before using California Poppy, especially if you are pregnant, breastfeeding, or taking other medications, as it may interact with certain substances.

California Poppy offers a natural way to relax and unwind. Its sedative and analgesic properties make it a valuable herb for promoting calmness, easing tension, and supporting overall well-being. If you are seeking a gentle and natural approach to relaxation, California Poppy may be a beneficial herb to incorporate into your daily routine.

SKULLCAP

Skullcap, also known as Scutellaria, is a medicinal plant that has been used for centuries in traditional herbal medicine. There are several species of Skullcap, including American Skullcap (Scutellaria lateriflora) and Chinese Skullcap (Scutellaria baicalensis), each with its own unique properties and health benefits.

One of the main ailments that Skullcap addresses is anxiety and stress. It has a calming effect on the nervous system and can help promote relaxation. Skullcap is often used as a natural remedy for anxiety, nervous tension, and insomnia. It may also help reduce symptoms of depression and improve overall mood.

Skullcap has also been used for its anti-inflammatory properties. Studies have shown that certain compounds found in Skullcap, such as baicalin and baicalein, possess anti-inflammatory effects. This makes it potentially beneficial for conditions like arthritis, inflammatory bowel disease, and other inflammatory conditions.

Skullcap has been traditionally used for its antispasmodic properties, which can help alleviate muscle spasms and cramps. It may be useful in managing conditions such as menstrual cramps or muscle tension.

In addition, Skullcap is sometimes used as a natural remedy for headaches and migraines. Its calming effects may help reduce the intensity and frequency of these headaches.

Please note that while Skullcap has been traditionally used for these purposes, it's essential to consult with a healthcare professional before using any herbal remedies, especially if you have any existing medical conditions or are taking medication. They can provide personalized guidance based on your specific situation.

LEMON BALM

Lemon Balm (Melissa officinalis) is a herb known for its medicinal properties and its pleasant lemony aroma. It has been used for centuries in traditional medicine to address various health issues. *Here are a few of the medicinal benefits associated with Lemon Balm:*

ANXIETY AND STRESS RELIEF:

Lemon Balm is well-known for its calming effects on the nervous system. It has been used as a natural remedy for anxiety, nervousness, and restlessness. Lemon Balm may help promote relaxation and reduce feelings of tension, making it beneficial for individuals dealing with mild anxiety or stress.

SLEEP AID:

Due to its calming properties, Lemon Balm is also used as a natural sleep aid. It may help improve sleep quality and duration, making it useful for those who struggle with insomnia or occasional sleep disturbances. Drinking Lemon Balm tea before bedtime is a popular way to promote relaxation and prepare the body for sleep.

DIGESTIVE SUPPORT:

Lemon Balm has been traditionally used to support digestive health. It may help relieve digestive discomfort, bloating, and flatulence. Additionally, Lemon Balm has a mild antispasmodic effect that can help reduce stomach cramps and spasms.

MOOD ENHANCEMENT:

Lemon Balm is known for its mood-lifting properties. It may help improve mood and reduce feelings of sadness or low spirits. Some studies suggest that Lemon Balm extracts may have positive effects on neurotransmitters in the brain, helping to improve mood and overall mental well-being.

COLD SORE TREATMENT:

Topical applications of Lemon Balm can be beneficial in treating cold sores caused by the herpes simplex virus. Lemon Balm extracts possess antiviral properties that may help reduce the duration and severity of cold sores when applied directly to the affected area.

It's important to note that while Lemon Balm is generally considered safe for most individuals, it's always a good idea to consult with a healthcare professional before using any herbal remedies, especially if you have any underlying health conditions or are taking medications that may interact with Lemon Balm.

ASIAN GINSENG

Asian Ginseng, also known as Panax ginseng, is a popular herb widely used in traditional Chinese medicine for its numerous medicinal benefits. *Here are a few of the medicinal benefits associated with Asian Ginseng:*

ENERGY AND STAMINA BOOST:

Asian Ginseng is often used as an adaptogen to combat fatigue and increase energy levels. It is believed to help enhance physical endurance and mental alertness. Regular consumption of Asian Ginseng may help improve overall energy and stamina levels, making it beneficial for individuals dealing with fatigue or weakness.

COGNITIVE FUNCTION AND MENTAL CLARITY:

Asian Ginseng has been traditionally used for its potential cognitive-enhancing properties. It may help improve focus, memory, and overall mental performance. Some studies suggest that Asian Ginseng may have neuroprotective effects and could potentially help reduce age-related cognitive decline.

STRESS AND IMMUNE SUPPORT:

Asian Ginseng is known for its adaptogenic properties, meaning it may help the body better cope with stress and support a healthy immune system. It is believed to help regulate the stress hormone cortisol and support overall immune function. Regular intake of Asian Ginseng may help strengthen the body's resilience against stressors and promote overall well-being.

BLOOD SUGAR REGULATION:

Asian Ginseng may have potential benefits for individuals with diabetes or those at risk of developing the condition. Some studies suggest that Asian Ginseng may help regulate blood sugar levels by improving insulin sensitivity. However, it's important to note that Asian Ginseng should not replace standard diabetes treatments, and consulting with a healthcare professional is crucial for managing blood sugar levels.

SEXUAL HEALTH:

Asian Ginseng has long been used as an aphrodisiac and sexual tonic. It is believed to help improve libido and sexual function in both men and women. Some studies suggest that Asian Ginseng may help increase testosterone levels in men, leading to improved sexual performance.

**It's essential to remember that Asian Ginseng may interact with certain medications and may not be suitable for everyone. It's best to consult with a healthcare professional before incorporating Asian Ginseng into your routine, especially if you have any underlying health conditions or take medications.**

GOTU KOLA

Gotu kola, also known as Centella asiatica, is a herb traditionally used in Ayurvedic and traditional Chinese medicine for its various health benefits. *Here are a few medicinal benefits associated with gotu kola:*

COGNITIVE FUNCTION:

Gotu kola has been used for centuries as a brain tonic and is believed to improve cognitive function. It is thought to enhance memory, concentration, and overall mental clarity. Some studies suggest that gotu kola may stimulate the production of new brain cells, potentially benefiting individuals dealing with age-related cognitive decline.

WOUND HEALING:

Gotu kola is known for its wound-healing properties. It is believed to enhance the synthesis of collagen, a protein essential for maintaining the structure and elasticity of the skin. Regular application of gotu kola topically or consumption of supplements may help improve the healing of wounds, cuts, and scars.

ANXIETY AND STRESS RELIEF:

Gotu kola is often regarded as an adaptogen, a substance that helps the body adapt to physical and emotional stress. It is believed to have a calming and relaxing effect on the nervous system, potentially reducing anxiety and stress levels. Some studies suggest that gotu kola may help balance stress hormones, such as cortisol.

SKIN HEALTH:

Gotu kola is commonly used in skincare products due to its potential benefits for the skin. It is believed to help improve skin tone and texture, reduce the appearance of scars and stretch marks, and promote overall skin health. Gotu kola may also have antioxidant properties that help protect the skin from free radical damage.

VARICOSE VEINS AND CIRCULATION:

Gotu kola is traditionally used to support healthy circulation and to alleviate symptoms of venous insufficiency, such as varicose veins and swelling. It is believed to strengthen the walls of blood vessels and improve blood flow, potentially reducing the occurrence and severity of varicose veins.

**It's important to note that while gotu kola is generally considered safe, it may interact with certain medications or have contraindications for certain individuals. Always consult with a healthcare professional before incorporating gotu kola into your routine, especially if you have any underlying health conditions or take medications.**

<u>HOLY BASIL</u>

Sure! Holy Basil, also known as Tulsi or Ocimum sanctum, is a sacred herb in Ayurveda with a wide range of medicinal benefits. ***Here are a few of its key medicinal properties and uses:***

ADAPTOGENIC PROPERTIES:

Holy Basil is classified as an adaptogen, meaning it helps the body adapt to various stressors and restore balance. It is believed to have a positive impact on the adrenal glands, reducing stress and anxiety while promoting relaxation and mental clarity.

ANTIOXIDANT AND ANTI-INFLAMMATORY EFFECTS:

Holy Basil contains phytochemicals that act as antioxidants, protecting the body from damage caused by harmful free radicals. It also has anti-inflammatory properties, which may help reduce inflammation in the body and alleviate symptoms of chronic conditions like arthritis.

RESPIRATORY HEALTH:

Holy Basil has been used for centuries as a natural remedy for respiratory ailments. It is believed to help relieve symptoms of cough, cold, and respiratory infections by soothing irritated airways and reducing inflammation. It may also have expectorant properties that help expel mucus from the lungs.

DIGESTIVE AID:

Holy Basil is often used to support digestive health. It is believed to help relieve digestive issues such as bloating, indigestion, and stomach cramps. Holy Basil may also promote healthy gut bacteria and improve overall gut health.

IMMUNE BOOSTER:

Holy Basil is rich in antioxidants and essential oils that help strengthen the immune system. Regular consumption of Holy Basil tea or supplements may help boost immunity and protect against common infections.

HORMONAL BALANCE:

Holy Basil is believed to have a positive effect on hormone levels, particularly those related to stress and reproductive health. It may help regulate cortisol levels, reducing stress-related symptoms. Additionally, Holy Basil may have a balancing effect on female hormones, potentially relieving symptoms of hormonal imbalances such as PMS.

It's important to note that while Holy Basil is generally considered safe, it may interact with certain medications or have contraindications for certain individuals. Always consult with a healthcare professional before incorporating Holy Basil into your routine, especially if you have any underlying health conditions or take medications.

LAVENDER

Lavender is a versatile herb that has been used for centuries for its various medicinal benefits. It is well-known for its calming and soothing properties, making it a popular choice in aromatherapy and alternative medicine. *Here are a few of its medicinal benefits:*

RELAXATION AND STRESS RELIEF:

The aroma of lavender has been shown to promote relaxation and reduce stress levels. It can help calm the nervous system, ease anxiety, and improve sleep quality. Many people use lavender essential oil or enjoy a warm lavender bath to unwind and de-stress.

HEADACHE RELIEF:

Lavender has analgesic properties that can help alleviate tension headaches and migraines. Applying diluted lavender oil to the temples or inhaling its aroma may provide relief from headache symptoms.

SKIN CARE:

Lavender has anti-inflammatory and antiseptic properties, making it beneficial for various skin conditions. It can help soothe skin irritations, rashes, and minor burns. Lavender oil is commonly used in skincare products like lotions, creams, and soaps.

DIGESTIVE HEALTH:

Lavender has been used to aid digestion and soothe stomach discomfort. It can help relieve bloating, indigestion, and flatulence. Drinking lavender tea or using lavender oil in a massage blend on the abdomen may provide relief.

PAIN RELIEF:

Lavender has mild analgesic properties that can help alleviate muscle aches, joint pain, and minor injuries. Applying lavender oil topically or using it in a warm compress can help reduce pain and inflammation.

**It's important to note that while lavender is generally considered safe for most people, some individuals may experience allergic reactions or skin sensitivities. It's always a good idea to do a patch test before using lavender oil topically, and consult with a healthcare professional if you have any specific health concerns or conditions.**

FENNEL

Fennel is a herb commonly used in cooking, and it also offers various medicinal benefits. ***Here are some of the ailments fennel can address and its medicinal benefits:***

DIGESTIVE ISSUES:

Fennel has been used for centuries to treat digestive ailments. It can help relieve bloating, gas, and indigestion. Fennel seeds contain compounds that stimulate digestion and help relax the muscles of the gastrointestinal tract, promoting better digestion and reducing discomfort.

MENSTRUAL CRAMPS:

Fennel can help alleviate menstrual cramps and other symptoms associated with PMS (premenstrual syndrome). It has antispasmodic properties that can help relax the muscles in the uterus and reduce pain.

RESPIRATORY CONDITIONS:

Fennel has been used traditionally to relieve respiratory conditions such as coughs and bronchitis. It has expectorant properties, which means it helps loosen mucus and phlegm, making it easier to cough up and clear the airways.

EYE HEALTH:

Fennel contains antioxidants and vitamins that are beneficial for eye health. It can help reduce inflammation in the eyes and provide relief from conditions like conjunctivitis and eye strain.

GENERAL WELLNESS:

Fennel is rich in antioxidants and has anti-inflammatory properties, which can contribute to overall health and well-being. It may help boost the immune system, reduce inflammation in the body, and protect against chronic diseases.

**It's worth noting that while fennel is generally safe for most people, it may interact with certain medications or cause allergic reactions in some individuals. If you have any specific health concerns or conditions, it's always a good idea to consult with a healthcare professional before using fennel medicinally.**

CALENDULA

Calendula, also known as marigold, is a vibrant flower that offers various medicinal benefits. It has been used for centuries for its healing properties. ***Here are some of the ailments that calendula can address and its medicinal benefits:***

SKIN CONDITIONS:

Calendula is widely known for its soothing and healing effects on the skin. It can be used to alleviate various skin conditions, including rashes, eczema, dermatitis, and minor cuts, burns, and wounds. Calendula has anti-inflammatory and antimicrobial properties that help reduce redness, inflammation, and promote skin regeneration.

WOUND HEALING:

Due to its antibacterial and antifungal properties, calendula can aid in wound healing. It helps to protect the wound from infection and promotes faster healing. Calendula oil or ointment can be applied topically to cuts, scrapes, and minor burns.

SKIN REJUVENATION:

Regular use of calendula-infused products can promote healthier and rejuvenated skin. Calendula extracts are often used in skincare products due to their ability to improve skin hydration, reduce signs of aging, and promote a more youthful complexion.

MENSTRUAL CRAMPS:

Calendula is believed to have antispasmodic properties, which can help relax the muscles and alleviate menstrual cramps. Drinking calendula tea during menstruation may provide relief from cramps and discomfort.

DIGESTIVE HEALTH:

Calendula has been traditionally used to support digestive health. It can stimulate the production of digestive juices, improve digestion, and reduce symptoms of indigestion and bloating. Calendula tea or tinctures can be consumed to support digestive wellness.

It's important to note that while calendula is generally considered safe for most people when used topically or internally in moderation, allergic reactions can occur in some individuals. If you have any specific health concerns or conditions, it's advisable to consult with a healthcare professional before using calendula medicinally.

EUCALYPTUS

Eucalyptus is a type of tree that is widely recognized for its medicinal properties. It has been used for centuries for various ailments and offers numerous health benefits. ***Here are some of the ailments that eucalyptus can address and its medicinal benefits:***

RESPIRATORY CONDITIONS:

Eucalyptus is known for its ability to alleviate respiratory problems. The leaves contain a compound called cineole, which has expectorant and decongestant properties. Eucalyptus oil or inhalation of eucalyptus steam can help relieve symptoms of coughs, colds, sinus congestion, bronchitis, and even asthma.

SORE THROAT AND COUGH:

Eucalyptus can provide relief for sore throats and coughs. Gargling with eucalyptus-infused water or using throat lozenges with eucalyptus can soothe throat irritation and suppress coughing.

PAIN RELIEF:

Eucalyptus oil has analgesic properties that can help numb pain and reduce inflammation. It is often used topically to relieve muscle and joint pain, headaches, and arthritis. Massage oils or balms containing eucalyptus can be applied to the affected area for relief.

SKIN INFECTIONS:

Eucalyptus oil possesses antimicrobial and antiseptic properties, making it effective in treating skin infections and promoting wound healing. It can be used topically to cleanse and protect cuts, burns, and insect bites.

MENTAL CLARITY AND RELAXATION:

The aroma of eucalyptus has refreshing and invigorating effects on the mind. It can help improve concentration, boost mental clarity, and alleviate mental fatigue. Inhalation of eucalyptus oil or using it in aromatherapy diffusers can promote relaxation and a sense of well-being.

**Eucalyptus is generally safe for most individuals when used appropriately. However, it's important to note that pure eucalyptus oil can be toxic if ingested in large amounts or used directly on the skin without dilution. It is always recommended to follow proper usage guidelines and consult with a healthcare professional if you have any specific health concerns or conditions.**

PEPPERMINT

Peppermint is a popular herb that provides a range of health benefits. ***Here are some common ailments that peppermint can address and its medicinal benefits:***

DIGESTIVE ISSUES:

Peppermint is well-known for its ability to soothe digestive discomfort. It can help relieve symptoms of indigestion, bloating, gas, and stomach cramps. Peppermint oil works by relaxing the muscles of the gastrointestinal tract, promoting smoother digestion.

HEADACHES AND MIGRAINES:

Peppermint contains menthol, which has a cooling effect and can help alleviate tension headaches and migraines. Applying diluted peppermint oil to the temples or inhaling its aroma may provide relief.

RESPIRATORY CONDITIONS:

Peppermint has decongestant and expectorant properties, making it effective in relieving respiratory issues. It can help with symptoms of coughs, congestion, sinusitis, and asthma. Drinking peppermint tea or inhaling peppermint steam can provide relief.

MUSCLE PAIN AND TENSION:

The cooling effect of peppermint is also beneficial for relieving muscle pain, tension, and soreness. Applying a diluted peppermint oil or using a peppermint-infused massage oil can help relax muscles and reduce discomfort.

MENTAL ALERTNESS:

The aroma of peppermint has an invigorating effect, promoting mental clarity and alertness. It can help improve focus, concentration, and memory. Inhaling peppermint essential oil or using it in a diffuser can enhance cognitive performance.

NAUSEA AND MOTION SICKNESS:

Peppermint has been traditionally used to alleviate nausea and motion sickness. Drinking peppermint tea or using peppermint essential oil in a diffuser can help calm an upset stomach.

**It's worth noting that while peppermint is generally safe for most people, it may cause allergic reactions or interact with certain medications in some individuals. Additionally, undiluted or excessive use of peppermint oil can irritate the skin or mucous membranes. It's best to consult with a healthcare professional before using peppermint for any specific health concerns or if you have underlying medical conditions.**

<u>GINKO BILBOA</u>

Ginkgo Biloba is an herbal supplement derived from the leaves of the Ginkgo Biloba tree. It has been used for centuries in traditional Chinese medicine and is believed to offer several health benefits. *Here are some common ailments that Ginkgo Biloba may address and its associated medicinal benefits:*

COGNITIVE FUNCTION AND MEMORY:

Ginkgo Biloba is frequently used to support cognitive health and enhance memory. It is thought to improve blood circulation to the brain, which may help boost memory, concentration, and overall cognitive function.

AGE-RELATED COGNITIVE DECLINE:

It is believed that Ginkgo Biloba may help slow down or reduce age-related cognitive decline, including conditions such as dementia and Alzheimer's disease. However, more research is needed to fully understand its effectiveness in this regard.

EYE HEALTH:

Ginkgo Biloba may have positive effects on eye health by increasing blood flow and protecting retinal cells from damage. It is believed to support vision and may be beneficial in managing conditions such as macular degeneration and glaucoma, although further research is required.

TINNITUS:

Tinnitus refers to a ringing or buzzing sound in the ears. Ginkgo Biloba has been suggested as a potential treatment for tinnitus due to its ability to improve blood flow and reduce inflammation. Some individuals have reported experiencing relief from their tinnitus symptoms with the use of Ginkgo Biloba, but the results vary.

PERIPHERAL ARTERY DISEASE:

Ginkgo Biloba may aid in managing symptoms of peripheral artery disease (PAD) by improving blood circulation and reducing inflammation. PAD is a condition characterized by narrowed or blocked blood vessels, mainly affecting the legs. However, it's essential to consult with a healthcare professional before using Ginkgo Biloba to manage any medical condition.

ANXIETY AND DEPRESSION:

Some studies have suggested that Ginkgo Biloba may have potential benefits for anxiety and depression. It may help reduce symptoms and improve mood, but more research is needed to establish its effectiveness and safety in treating these conditions.

It's important to note that individual results and the effectiveness of Ginkgo Biloba can vary. Ginkgo Biloba may interact with certain medications or have side effects, so it's crucial to consult with a healthcare professional before using it, especially if you have any underlying health conditions or take other medications.

<u>VITEX</u>

Vitex, also known as Chaste Tree or Chasteberry, is a flowering plant that has been used for centuries in traditional herbal medicine. It is frequently used to address hormonal imbalances in women and may offer several medicinal benefits. ***Here are some common ailments that Vitex may address and its associated medicinal benefits:***

MENSTRUAL DISORDERS:

Vitex is often used to regulate menstrual cycles, especially in cases of irregular or absent periods. It can help balance hormone levels and may alleviate symptoms like menstrual cramps, breast tenderness, and mood swings. Vitex is commonly used by women experiencing premenstrual syndrome (PMS) and may help in managing the symptoms.

INFERTILITY AND FERTILITY SUPPORT:

Vitex has been used for reproductive health and fertility support. It may help regulate ovulation, improve luteal phase defects, and support overall reproductive function. However, it is important to note that individual responses to Vitex may vary, and it is recommended to consult with a healthcare professional, especially for fertility concerns.

MENOPAUSE SYMPTOMS:

Vitex may help alleviate symptoms associated with menopause, such as hot flashes, night sweats, mood swings, and sleep disturbances. It is believed to have an estrogen-like effect and can help balance hormone levels during this transitional phase.

ACNE AND SKIN ISSUES:

Vitex has anti-androgenic properties, meaning it may help reduce the production of male hormones (androgens) in the body. This hormonal regulation may be beneficial for individuals experiencing hormonal acne or other skin issues related to hormonal imbalances.

BREAST PAIN:

Vitex is known for its potential to reduce breast pain and tenderness associated with fibrocystic breasts. It may help regulate fluid retention in breast tissue and alleviate discomfort.

MOOD AND ANXIETY:

Vitex is believed to have mood-stabilizing effects and may promote emotional well-being. It is commonly used to address symptoms of anxiety, irritability, and mood swings associated with hormonal imbalances.

It is important to note that Vitex may take time to show its effects, and individual responses may vary. It is generally considered safe for consumption but may interact with certain medications or hormone therapies. As always, it is recommended to consult with a healthcare professional before incorporating Vitex into your routine, especially if you have any underlying health conditions or take prescription medications.

BLACK COHOSH

Black Cohosh, also known as Actaea racemosa, is a herbaceous plant that has been traditionally used for its medicinal properties. *Here are some common ailments that Black Cohosh may address and its associated medicinal benefits:*

MENOPAUSE SYMPTOMS:

Black Cohosh is perhaps best known for its use in alleviating symptoms associated with menopause. It is believed to have estrogen-like effects and is commonly used to reduce hot flashes, night sweats, and mood swings. The herb may also support a better sleep pattern during menopause.

PREMENSTRUAL SYNDROME (PMS):

Black Cohosh may help in managing the symptoms of PMS, such as irritability, bloating, breast tenderness, and mood swings. It is thought to have mood-stabilizing properties and may alleviate these symptoms.

MENSTRUAL IRREGULARITIES:

Some women experience irregular periods, and Black Cohosh may help regulate menstrual cycles. It may aid in establishing a more regular pattern by balancing hormone levels.

OSTEOPOROSIS:

Black Cohosh is believed to have bone-protective effects and may help in maintaining bone health. It may support the prevention of osteoporosis, a condition characterized by decreased bone density and increased risk of fractures.

MOOD DISORDERS:

Black Cohosh is sometimes used as a natural remedy for mood disorders such as anxiety and depression. It may have an anti-anxiety effect and help in reducing stress levels.

RHEUMATOID ARTHRITIS:

Black Cohosh has been used traditionally to alleviate symptoms of rheumatoid arthritis, including joint pain and inflammation. It may have anti-inflammatory properties and could potentially provide some relief.

It's important to note that while Black Cohosh may offer some benefits, individual responses can vary, and it may interact with certain medications or have contraindications for specific health conditions. It is advisable to consult with a healthcare professional before starting any new herbal supplement or remedy. They will be able to provide personalized advice based on your specific circumstances.

DONG QUAI

Dong Quai, also known as Angelica sinensis or "female ginseng," is a herb that has been used in traditional Chinese medicine for centuries. *It is believed to have various medicinal benefits and is commonly used to address the following ailments:*

MENSTRUAL DISORDERS:

Dong Quai is frequently used to regulate and promote a healthy menstrual cycle. It may help alleviate symptoms of menstrual cramps, irregular periods, and excessive bleeding. It is often used as a natural remedy for conditions like dysmenorrhea and menorrhagia.

MENOPAUSAL SYMPTOMS:

Similar to Black Cohosh, Dong Quai may support women experiencing menopausal symptoms such as hot flashes, mood swings, and vaginal dryness. It is believed to have estrogen-like effects and may help rebalance hormone levels during this transitional period.

PAIN RELIEF:

Dong Quai is known for its analgesic and anti-inflammatory properties. It may help reduce pain associated with headaches, migraines, and muscle cramps. It is often used as a natural alternative to nonsteroidal anti-inflammatory drugs (NSAIDs).

BLOOD CIRCULATION:

Dong Quai is believed to have vasodilatory effects, which means it may promote healthy blood flow and circulation. This may be beneficial for conditions like Raynaud's disease and other circulatory disorders.

STRESS AND ANXIETY:

Dong Quai has been traditionally used as an adaptogen, which means it can help the body cope with stressors. It may have a calming effect on the nervous system and be beneficial in reducing anxiety and promoting overall relaxation.

DIGESTIVE HEALTH:

Dong Quai has been used to support digestive health and relieve symptoms of gastrointestinal issues such as bloating, indigestion, and constipation. It may have mild laxative properties and help improve overall gut function.

Dong Quai is available in various forms, including capsules, tinctures, and teas. As with any herbal remedy, it's important to consult with a healthcare professional before starting a new supplement, especially if you have any existing health conditions or are taking medications. They can provide personalized advice based on your specific needs.

<u>TURMERIC</u>

Turmeric, scientifically known as Curcuma longa, is a yellow-colored spice commonly used in cooking. It has been extensively studied for its medicinal properties and contains a compound called curcumin that gives it its vibrant color and many of its health benefits. ***Here are a few of the medicinal benefits associated with turmeric:***

ANTI-INFLAMMATORY PROPERTIES:

Curcumin, the active compound in turmeric, has powerful anti-inflammatory effects. It can help reduce chronic inflammation, which is believed to be the root cause of many diseases, including heart disease, cancer, and arthritis.

ANTIOXIDANT ACTIVITY:

Turmeric contains potent antioxidants that can neutralize harmful free radicals in the body. This antioxidant activity may help protect against oxidative damage and reduce the risk of chronic diseases.

PAIN RELIEF:

Turmeric has been used for centuries in traditional medicine as a natural pain reliever. It may help alleviate pain associated with conditions like osteoarthritis, rheumatoid arthritis, and general muscle or joint pain.

DIGESTIVE HEALTH:

Turmeric has been used to support digestion and alleviate symptoms of gastrointestinal disorders. It may promote the production of digestive enzymes, reduce bloating and gas, and even help with conditions like irritable bowel syndrome (IBS).

BRAIN HEALTH:

Some studies suggest that curcumin may have neuroprotective properties and could potentially help prevent or delay brain-related diseases such as Alzheimer's disease and Parkinson's disease. It is believed to cross the blood-brain barrier and have anti-inflammatory and antioxidant effects in the brain.

HEART HEALTH:

Turmeric may have beneficial effects on heart health. It may help improve the function of the endothelium, the lining of blood vessels, and reduce the risk of heart disease by improving cholesterol levels, decreasing blood clot formation, and reducing inflammation.

SKIN HEALTH:

Turmeric is used in various skincare products due to its potential benefits for the skin. It may help reduce inflammation, acne, and even lighten pigmentation or scars when used topically.

It is important to note that while turmeric has many potential health benefits, its medicinal effects can vary depending on factors such as the dosage, bioavailability, and individual response. It is commonly consumed as a spice in cooking, but for therapeutic purposes, higher doses may be required. Curcumin supplements are also available, often combined with other ingredients to enhance its absorption.

ALOE VERA

Aloe vera is a succulent plant that has been used for thousands of years for its medicinal and healing properties. It is known for its gel-like substance found in its leaves, which contains an array of beneficial compounds. ***Here are a few of its medicinal benefits:***

SKIN HEALTH:

Aloe vera is most commonly associated with its benefits for skin health. It has soothing and moisturizing properties that can help alleviate various skin conditions such as sunburns, rashes, eczema, psoriasis, and acne. It may also aid in wound healing and reduce scarring.

ANTI-INFLAMMATORY EFFECTS:

Aloe vera contains compounds, including vitamins, enzymes, and minerals, that have anti-inflammatory properties. When applied topically or consumed internally, it may help reduce inflammation in the body and alleviate symptoms of conditions such as arthritis and inflammatory bowel disease.

DIGESTIVE SUPPORT:

Aloe vera has been used as a natural remedy for digestive issues such as constipation and irritable bowel syndrome (IBS). It contains compounds that can help improve digestion, promote bowel movements, and soothe gastrointestinal discomfort.

IMMUNE SYSTEM SUPPORT:

Aloe vera is rich in antioxidants, which can help boost the immune system and protect the body against harmful free radicals. It may also have antimicrobial properties, potentially aiding in the prevention and treatment of infections.

ORAL HEALTH:

Aloe vera gel can be used as a natural mouthwash or added to toothpaste due to its potential benefits for oral health. It may help reduce plaque buildup, fight against bacteria that cause gum disease, and alleviate mouth ulcers or sores.

DIABETES MANAGEMENT:

Some studies suggest that aloe vera may have beneficial effects on blood sugar control. It may help improve insulin sensitivity and reduce fasting blood sugar levels in individuals with prediabetes or type 2 diabetes. However, more research is needed in this area.

ANTICANCER PROPERTIES:

Preliminary research has shown that certain compounds found in aloe vera may have anticancer effects. They may help inhibit the growth of cancer cells and induce cell death. However, further studies are necessary to fully understand its potential in cancer prevention and treatment.

It is important to note that while aloe vera is generally considered safe when used appropriately, it may cause allergic reactions or skin irritation in some individuals. It is always recommended to do a patch test before applying it to a larger area of the skin and to

consult with a healthcare professional if you have any underlying health conditions or are taking medications.

Additionally, it is crucial to use aloe vera products that are of high quality and free from additives or contaminants. This can ensure that you are receiving the maximum benefits from the plant.

CHAPTER 4

IMMUNE BOOST TINCTURE (OPTION 1):

INGREDIENTS:

Reishi, Lion's Mane, Cordyceps, Turkey Tail, Elderberries, Echinacea

PREPARATION:

Mix equal parts of dried Reishi, Lion's Mane, Cordyceps, and Turkey Tail mushrooms with elderberries and echinacea. Finely chop or grind the ingredients. Place the mixture in a glass jar and cover with alcohol, such as vodka or brandy. Seal the jar tightly and store in a cool, dark place for 4-6 weeks, shaking daily. Strain the tincture and store in a labeled amber glass dropper bottle.

BENEFITS:

This tincture helps boost the immune system, supports respiratory health, and offers antiviral and antibacterial properties.

STORAGE:

Store the jar in a cool, dark place. After 4-6 weeks, strain the tincture using cheesecloth or a fine-mesh strainer, and transfer the liquid into amber glass dropper bottles for easy use. This tincture can be stored for up to 5 years.

<u>**IMMUNE BOOST TINCTURE (OPTION 2):**</u>

<u>*INGREDIENTS:*</u>

Reishi, Echinacea, Elderberries, Licorice Root, Ginger

<u>*PREPARATION:*</u>

Combine equal parts of the dried herbs in a glass jar. Cover with alcohol (such as vodka) and let it steep for 4-6 weeks, shaking the jar regularly. Strain and store in a dark glass bottle.

<u>*STORAGE:*</u>

Store in a cool, dark place. Store the jar in a cool, dark place. After 4-6 weeks, strain the tincture using cheesecloth or a fine-mesh strainer, and transfer the liquid into amber glass dropper bottles for easy use. This tincture can be stored for up to 5 years.

IMMUNE SUPPORT TINCTURE:

INGREDIENTS:

Reishi, Lions Mane, Cordyceps, Turkey Tail, Elderberries, Echinacea.

PREPARATION:

Combine equal parts of each herb (e.g., 1 ounce or 30 grams each) in a glass jar. Cover them with vodka or another high-proof alcohol, ensuring all the herbs are submerged. Seal the jar tightly.

STORAGE:

Store the jar in a cool, dark place. After 4-6 weeks, strain the tincture using cheesecloth or a fine-mesh strainer, and transfer the liquid into amber glass dropper bottles for easy use. This tincture can be stored for up to 5 years.

<u>**COGNITIVE FUNCTION TINCTURE:**</u>

<u>*INGREDIENTS:*</u>

Lions Mane, Ginkgo Biloba, Rosemary, Tulsi, Ginger

<u>*PREPARATION:*</u>

Combine equal parts of the dried herbs in a glass jar. Cover with alcohol and let it steep for 4-6 weeks, shaking the jar regularly. Strain and store in a dark glass bottle.

<u>*STORAGE:*</u>

Store in a cool, dark place. After 4-6 weeks, strain the tincture using cheesecloth or a fine-mesh strainer, and transfer the liquid into amber glass dropper bottles for easy use. This tincture can be stored for up to 5 years.

<u>**ANTI-INFLAMMATORY TINCTURE:**</u>

<u>*INGREDIENTS:*</u>

Turmeric, Ginger, Meadowsweet, Holy Basil, Licorice Root

<u>*PREPARATION:*</u>

Combine equal parts of the dried herbs in a glass jar. Cover with alcohol and let it steep for 4-6 weeks, shaking the jar regularly. Strain and store in a dark glass bottle.

<u>*STORAGE:*</u>

Store in a cool, dark place. After 4-6 weeks, strain the tincture using cheesecloth or a fine-mesh strainer, and transfer the liquid into amber glass dropper bottles for easy use. This tincture can be stored for up to 5 years.

DIGESTIVE SUPPORT TINCTURE (OPTION 1):

INGREDIENTS:

Ginger, Licorice Root, Meadowsweet

PREPARATION:

Mix equal parts of dried ginger, licorice root, and meadowsweet. Finely chop or grind the ingredients. Place the mixture in a glass jar and cover with alcohol. Seal the jar tightly and store in a cool, dark place for 4-6 weeks, shaking daily. Strain the tincture and store in a labeled amber glass dropper bottle.

STORAGE:

Store in a cool, dark place. After 4-6 weeks, strain the tincture using cheesecloth or a fine-mesh strainer, and transfer the liquid into amber glass dropper bottles for easy use. This tincture can be stored for up to 5 years.

BENEFITS:

This tincture aids digestion, reduces inflammation, soothes stomach discomfort, and supports overall digestive health.

DIGESTIVE SUPPORT TINCTURE (OPTION 2):

INGREDIENTS:

Dandelion, Burdock, Fennel, Ginger, Calendula

PREPARATION:

Combine equal parts of the dried herbs in a glass jar. Cover with alcohol and let it steep for 4-6 weeks, shaking the jar regularly. Strain and store in a dark glass bottle.

STORAGE:

Store in a cool, dark place. After 4-6 weeks, strain the tincture using cheesecloth or a fine-mesh strainer, and transfer the liquid into amber glass dropper bottles for easy use. This tincture can be stored for up to 5 years.

<u>DIGESTIVE HEALTH TINCTURE:</u>

<u>INGREDIENTS:</u>

Nettle, Ginger, Dandelion, Licorice Root, Meadowsweet, Chamomile.

<u>PREPARATION:</u>

Combine equal parts of each herb (e.g., 1 ounce or 30 grams each) in a glass jar. Cover them with vodka or another high-proof alcohol, ensuring all the herbs are submerged. Seal the jar tightly.

Shake the jar daily for 4-6 weeks to allow the alcohol to extract the medicinal compounds.

<u>STORAGE:</u>

Store the jar in a cool, dark place. After 4-6 weeks, strain the tincture using cheesecloth or a fine-mesh strainer, and transfer the liquid into amber glass dropper bottles for easy use. This tincture can be stored for up to 5 years.

<u>Remember to label your tinctures with the ingredients and date of preparation. Start with small doses (e.g., a dropperful) and gradually increase if needed.</u>

<u>**NERVINE RELAXATION TINCTURE:**</u>

<u>***INGREDIENTS:***</u>

Chamomile, Rose, Dandelion, Passion Flower, California Poppy

<u>***PREPARATION:***</u>

Mix equal parts of dried chamomile, rose petals, dandelion root, passion flower, and California poppy. Finely chop or grind the ingredients. Place the mixture in a glass jar and cover with alcohol. Seal the jar tightly and store in a cool, dark place for 4-6 weeks, shaking daily. Strain the tincture and store in a labeled amber glass dropper bottle.

<u>***STORAGE:***</u>

Store the jar in a cool, dark place. After 4-6 weeks, strain the tincture using cheesecloth or a fine-mesh strainer, and transfer the liquid into amber glass dropper bottles for easy use. This tincture can be stored for up to 5 years.

<u>***BENEFITS:***</u>

This tincture promotes relaxation, reduces anxiety, aids restful sleep, and helps relieve minor nervous tension.

<u>**NERVE SUPPORT TINCTURE:**</u>

INGREDIENTS:

1 part lion's mane mushrooms, 1 part St. John's Wort, 2 parts vodka or other high-proof alcohol.

PREPARATION:

Combine the lion's mane mushrooms and St. John's Wort in a glass jar. Add alcohol to cover the herbs completely. Seal the jar and let it sit for 4-6 weeks, shaking daily. Strain the tincture, and store it in a dark glass bottle.

STORAGE:

Store the jar in a cool, dark place. After 4-6 weeks, strain the tincture using cheesecloth or a fine-mesh strainer, and transfer the liquid into amber glass dropper bottles for easy use. This tincture can be stored for up to 5 years.

BENEFITS:

This tincture combines lion's mane mushrooms, known for their potential cognitive benefits, and St. John's Wort, which is traditionally used to support the nervous system.

NERVOUS SYSTEM TONIC TINCTURE:

INGREDIENTS:

Passion Flower, St. John's Wort, California Poppy, Skullcap, Lemon Balm

PREPARATION:

Combine equal parts of the dried herbs in a glass jar. Cover with alcohol and let it steep for 4-6 weeks, shaking the jar regularly. Strain and store in a dark glass bottle.

STORAGE:

Store in a cool, dark place. After 4-6 weeks, strain the tincture using cheesecloth or a fine-mesh strainer, and transfer the liquid into amber glass dropper bottles for easy use. This tincture can be stored for up to 5 years.

RESPIRATORY SUPPORT TINCTURE (OPTION 1):

INGREDIENTS:

Mullein, Thyme, Rosemary

PREPARATION:

Mix equal parts of dried mullein leaves, thyme, and rosemary. Finely chop or grind the ingredients. Place the mixture in a glass jar and cover with alcohol. Seal the jar tightly and store in a cool, dark place for 4-6 weeks, shaking daily. Strain the tincture and store in a labeled amber glass dropper bottle.

STORAGE:

Store in a cool, dark place. After 4-6 weeks, strain the tincture using cheesecloth or a fine-mesh strainer, and transfer the liquid into amber glass dropper bottles for easy use. This tincture can be stored for up to 5 years.

BENEFITS:

This tincture supports respiratory health, eases coughs, promotes clear breathing, and helps soothe throat irritation.

INGREDIENTS:

Mullein, Thyme, Eucalyptus, Peppermint, Marshmallow Root

PREPARATION:

Combine equal parts of the dried herbs in a glass jar. Cover with alcohol and let it steep for 4-6 weeks, shaking the jar regularly. Strain and store in a dark glass bottle.

STORAGE:

Store in a cool, dark place. After 4-6 weeks, strain the tincture using cheesecloth or a fine-mesh strainer, and transfer the liquid into amber glass dropper bottles for easy use. This tincture can be stored for up to 5 years.

Remember to consult with a healthcare professional or herbalist before using these tinctures, especially if you have any underlying medical conditions or are taking medication. And always follow the recommended dosage instructions.

<u>**ENERGY BOOST TINCTURE (OPTION 1):**</u>

INGREDIENTS:

2 parts cordyceps mushrooms, 1 part licorice root, 1 part ashwagandha root, 4 parts vodka or other high-proof alcohol.

PREPARATION:

Place the cordyceps mushrooms, licorice root, and ashwagandha root in a glass jar. Cover the herbs with alcohol, seal the jar, and let it steep for 4-6 weeks. Shake the jar regularly. After straining, transfer the tincture to a dark glass bottle.

BENEFITS:

This tincture combines cordyceps mushrooms, which may help enhance energy and athletic performance, with licorice root and ashwagandha, traditionally used to support the adrenals and overall energy levels.

ENERGY BOOSTING TINCTURE (OPTION 2):

INGREDIENTS:

Cordyceps, Asian Ginseng, Gotu Kola, Nettle, Ginger

PREPARATION:

Combine equal parts of the dried herbs in a glass jar. Cover with alcohol and let it steep for 4-6 weeks, shaking the jar regularly. Strain and store in a dark glass bottle.

STORAGE:

Store in a cool, dark place. After 4-6 weeks, strain the tincture using cheesecloth or a fine-mesh strainer, and transfer the liquid into amber glass dropper bottles for easy use. This tincture can be stored for up to 5 years.

Creating alcohol tinctures can be a great way to extract and preserve the medicinal properties of various herbs and mushrooms.

<u>**STRESS & ANXIETY RELIEF TINCTURE:**</u>

<u>INGREDIENTS:</u>

Ashwagandha, Passion Flower, Chamomile, St. John's Wort, California Poppy.

<u>RECIPE:</u>

Combine equal parts of each herb (e.g., 1 ounce or 30 grams each) in a glass jar. Cover them with vodka or another high-proof alcohol, ensuring all the herbs are submerged. Seal the jar tightly.

<u>PREPARATION:</u>

Shake the jar daily for 4-6 weeks to allow the alcohol to extract the medicinal compounds.

<u>STORAGE:</u>

Store the jar in a cool, dark place. After 4-6 weeks, strain the tincture using cheesecloth or a fine-mesh strainer, and transfer the liquid into amber glass dropper bottles for easy use. This tincture can be stored for up to 5 years.

<u>**STRESS RELIEF TINCTURE:**</u>

INGREDIENTS:

Ashwagandha, Holy Basil, Skullcap, Lemon Balm, Lavender

PREPARATION:

Combine equal parts of the dried herbs in a glass jar. Cover with alcohol and let it steep for 4-6 weeks, shaking the jar regularly. Strain and store in a dark glass bottle.

STORAGE:

Store in a cool, dark place. After 4-6 weeks, strain the tincture using cheesecloth or a fine-mesh strainer, and transfer the liquid into amber glass dropper bottles for easy use. This tincture can be stored for up to 5 years.

HORMONAL BALANCE TINCTURE:

INGREDIENTS:

Raspberry Leaf, Licorice Root, Vitex, Black Cohosh, Dong Quai

PREPARATION:

Combine equal parts of the dried herbs in a glass jar. Cover with alcohol and let it steep for 4-6 weeks, shaking the jar regularly. Strain and store in a dark glass bottle.

STORAGE:

Store the jar in a cool, dark place. After 4-6 weeks, strain the tincture using cheesecloth or a fine-mesh strainer, and transfer the liquid into amber glass dropper bottles for easy use. This tincture can be stored for up to 5 years.

SKIN HEALING TINCTURE:

INGREDIENTS:

Calendula, Rose, Lavender, Aloe Vera, Chamomile

PREPARATION:

Combine equal parts of the dried herbs in a glass jar. Cover with alcohol and let it steep for 4-6 weeks, shaking the jar regularly. Strain and store in a dark glass bottle.

STORAGE:

Store the jar in a cool, dark place. After 4-6 weeks, strain the tincture using cheesecloth or a fine-mesh strainer, and transfer the liquid into amber glass dropper bottles for easy use. This tincture can be stored for up to 5 years.

CHAPTER 5

To maintain the potency and effectiveness of tinctures, it is important to store them properly. **Here are some recommended storage methods:**

KEEP IN A COOL, DARK PLACE:

Tinctures are sensitive to light and heat, which can degrade their potency over time. Store them in a cool and dark location, such as a pantry or cabinet, away from direct sunlight and sources of heat like stoves or radiators.

SEAL THE BOTTLE TIGHTLY:

Ensure that the bottle containing the tincture is tightly sealed to prevent air from entering. Oxygen exposure can cause the constituents of the tincture to break down and lose their effectiveness.

USE AMBER OR DARK GLASS BOTTLES:

Tinctures are commonly sold in amber or dark glass bottles, which help to protect them from light exposure. If you are transferring a tincture into another container, choose a dark glass bottle to maintain its potency.

AVOID MOISTURE AND HUMIDITY:

Moisture and humidity can affect the quality of tinctures. Keep them away from areas like bathrooms or kitchens where moisture levels tend to be higher.

LABEL AND DATE THE BOTTLE:

It's important to label the tincture bottle with the name of the herb and the date it was made or purchased. This helps in keeping track of the potency and shelf life.

FOLLOW RECOMMENDED EXPIRATION DATES:
Tinctures usually have a shelf life of several years if stored correctly. However, it is advisable to check the expiration date provided by the manufacturer or herbalist and discard the tincture if it has expired.

Following these storage methods will help maintain the potency and efficacy of tinctures, allowing you to fully enjoy their benefits over an extended period of time.

Dosage guidelines for medicinal tinctures may vary depending on the specific herb or plant used, the concentration of the tincture, and the individual's age, weight, and overall health. It is always best to consult with a healthcare professional or herbalist for personalized dosage recommendations. ***However, here are some general guidelines:***

START LOW AND GO SLOW:

When using medicinal tinctures, it's generally recommended to start with a low dose and gradually increase if needed. This allows you to gauge your body's response and determine the appropriate dosage for your specific needs.

FOLLOW THE INSTRUCTIONS:

If you are using a commercially prepared tincture, carefully read and follow the instructions provided by the manufacturer. They often provide recommended dosages for different ailments or age groups.

ADJUST FOR BODY WEIGHT AND AGE:

Dosages for tinctures may be adjusted based on body weight and age. Children and individuals with lower body weight often require lower doses, while adults with higher body weight may need higher doses. It's important to consult with a healthcare professional to determine the appropriate dosage for your situation.

CONSIDER THE STRENGTH OF THE TINCTURE:
Tinctures can have different strengths depending on the plant
material to alcohol ratio. Higher alcohol percentages typically
result in stronger tinctures. If you are making your own tincture,
consider the strength of the tincture and adjust the dosage
accordingly.

TAKE INTO ACCOUNT THE CONDITION BEING TREATED:
The dosage may vary depending on the specific ailment or
condition being treated. Some herbs may require higher doses
for certain conditions, while others may require lower doses.
Again, consulting with a healthcare professional or herbalist can
provide specific guidance.

Remember, these guidelines are general in nature, and it's always best
to seek professional advice to ensure safe and appropriate use of
medicinal tinctures.

CHAPTER 6

Some of the most common physical ailments among humans include:

COMMON COLD: A viral infection that affects the respiratory system.

HEADACHES: Commonly caused by tension, dehydration, or migraines.

BACK PAIN: Often caused by muscle strain, injury, or poor posture.

ALLERGIES: Immune system reactions to various substances.

DIGESTIVE DISORDERS: Such as acid reflux, irritable bowel syndrome (IBS), or constipation.

As for mental health ailments, here are a few common ones:

DEPRESSION: A mood disorder characterized by persistent sadness and loss of interest.

ANXIETY DISORDERS: Conditions such as generalized anxiety disorder (GAD), panic disorder, or phobias.

BIPOLAR DISORDER: A mood disorder marked by alternating periods of depression and mania.

ATTENTION-DEFICIT/HYPERACTIVITY DISORDER (ADHD): A neurodevelopmental disorder that affects concentration and impulse control.

<u>**SUBSTANCE ABUSE DISORDERS:**</u> Conditions in which individuals struggle with addiction to substances like drugs or alcohol.

<u>Please note that this is not an exhaustive list, and there are many other physical and mental ailments that people can experience. It's always important to seek professional medical advice for accurate diagnosis and treatment.</u>

<u>RECIPE 1 - IMMUNE SUPPORT:</u>

INGREDIENTS:

- 1 part dried Echinacea root
- 1 part dried Elderberry
- 1 part fresh Garlic cloves
- 1 part dried Ginger root
- 1 part dried Peppermint leaves
- 80-100 proof alcohol (such as vodka or rum)

INSTRUCTIONS:

1. Combine equal parts of each herb in a glass jar with a tight-fitting lid.

2. Fill the jar halfway with the herb mixture.

3. Pour enough alcohol over the herbs to completely cover them, making sure there is at least an inch or so of alcohol above the herb mixture.

4. Close the jar tightly and shake well to mix the ingredients.

5. Store the jar in a cool, dark place, and shake it daily for about 4-6 weeks.

6. After the steeping period, strain the tincture through a muslin cloth or a fine mesh strainer to remove the herb solids.

7. Transfer the tincture liquid into a glass dropper bottle for easy use.

8. Take 1-2 dropperfuls (about 30-60 drops) of the tincture in a small amount of water up to 4 times a day when experiencing cold symptoms.

<u>**RECIPE 2 - ELDERBERRY AND GINGER:**</u>

INGREDIENTS:

- 2 parts dried Elderberry

- 1 part dried Ginger root

- 80-100 proof alcohol

INSTRUCTIONS:

1. In a glass jar with a tight-fitting lid, combine the elderberry and ginger root in the desired ratio.

2. Fill the jar halfway with the herb mixture.

3. Pour enough alcohol over the herbs to fully cover them with an inch or so of alcohol above the herb mixture.

4. Seal the jar tightly and give it a good shake to mix the ingredients.

5. Place the jar in a cool, dark place, and shake it daily for about 4-6 weeks.

6. After the steeping period, strain the tincture through a muslin cloth or a fine mesh strainer to remove the herb solids.

7. Transfer the liquid into a glass dropper bottle.

8. Take 1-2 dropperfuls (about 30-60 drops) of the tincture in a small amount of water up to 4 times a day to support relief from cold symptoms.

<u>Remember to consult with a healthcare professional before using these tinctures, especially if you have any underlying health conditions, are taking medications, or are pregnant or breastfeeding.</u>

HEADACHES

PEPPERMINT AND LAVENDER:

INGREDIENTS:

- 2 parts dried Peppermint leaves

- 1 part dried Lavender flowers

- 80-100 proof alcohol

INSTRUCTIONS:

1. Combine the dried peppermint leaves and dried lavender flowers in a glass jar with a tight-fitting lid.

2. Fill the jar halfway with the herb mixture.

3. Pour enough alcohol over the herbs to fully cover them with an inch or so of alcohol above the herb mixture.

4. Seal the jar tightly and give it a good shake to mix the ingredients.

5. Store the jar in a cool, dark place, and shake it daily for about 4-6 weeks.

6. After the steeping period, strain the tincture through a muslin cloth or a fine mesh strainer to remove the herb solids.

7. Transfer the liquid into a glass dropper bottle.

8. Take 1-2 dropperfuls (about 30-60 drops) of the tincture in a small amount of water as needed for headaches.

<u>**WILLOW BARK AND FEVERFEW:**</u>

INGREDIENTS:

- 2 parts dried Willow Bark

- 1 part dried Feverfew leaves and flowers

- 80-100 proof alcohol

INSTRUCTIONS:

1. Combine the dried willow bark and dried feverfew leaves and flowers in a glass jar with a tight-fitting lid.

2. Fill the jar halfway with the herb mixture.

3. Pour enough alcohol over the herbs to fully cover them with an inch or so of alcohol above the herb mixture.

4. Seal the jar tightly and give it a good shake to mix the ingredients.

5. Store the jar in a cool, dark place, and shake it daily for about 4-6 weeks.

6. After the steeping period, strain the tincture through a muslin cloth or a fine mesh strainer to remove the herb solids.

7. Transfer the liquid into a glass dropper bottle.

8. Take 1-2 dropperfuls (about 30-60 drops) of the tincture in a small amount of water as needed for headaches.

**Remember to consult with a healthcare professional before using these tinctures, especially if you have any underlying health conditions, are taking medications, or are pregnant or breastfeeding.**

<u>ARNICA AND ST. JOHN'S WORT:</u>

INGREDIENTS:

- 2 parts dried Arnica flowers

- 1 part dried St. John's Wort leaves and flowers

- 80-100 proof alcohol

INSTRUCTIONS:

1. Combine the dried arnica flowers and dried St. John's Wort leaves and flowers in a glass jar with a tight-fitting lid.

2. Fill the jar halfway with the herb mixture.

3. Pour enough alcohol over the herbs to fully cover them with an inch or so of alcohol above the herb mixture.

4. Seal the jar tightly and give it a good shake to mix the ingredients.

5. Store the jar in a cool, dark place, and shake it daily for about 4-6 weeks.

6. After the steeping period, strain the tincture through a muslin cloth or a fine mesh strainer to remove the herb solids.

7. Transfer the liquid into a glass dropper bottle.

8. Take 1-2 dropperfuls (about 30-60 drops) of the tincture in a small amount of water as needed for back pain.

<u>**DEVIL'S CLAW AND WHITE WILLOW BARK:**</u>

INGREDIENTS:

- 2 parts dried Devil's Claw root

- 1 part dried White Willow Bark

- 80-100 proof alcohol

INSTRUCTIONS:

1. Combine the dried Devil's Claw root and dried White Willow Bark in a glass jar with a tight-fitting lid.

2. Fill the jar halfway with the herb mixture.

3. Pour enough alcohol over the herbs to fully cover them with an inch or so of alcohol above the herb mixture.

4. Seal the jar tightly and give it a good shake to mix the ingredients.

5. Store the jar in a cool, dark place, and shake it daily for about 4-6 weeks.

6. After the steeping period, strain the tincture through a muslin cloth or a fine mesh strainer to remove the herb solids.

7. Transfer the liquid into a glass dropper bottle.

8. Take 1-2 dropperfuls (about 30-60 drops) of the tincture in a small amount of water as needed for back pain.

<u>Remember to consult with a healthcare professional before using these tinctures, especially if you have any underlying health conditions, are taking medications, or are pregnant or breastfeeding.</u>

ALLERGIES

NETTLE AND EYEBRIGHT:

INGREDIENTS:

- 2 parts dried Nettle leaf
- 1 part dried Eyebright herb
- 80-100 proof alcohol

INSTRUCTIONS:

1. Combine the dried Nettle leaf and dried Eyebright herb in a glass jar with a tight-fitting lid.

2. Fill the jar halfway with the herb mixture.

3. Pour enough alcohol over the herbs to fully cover them with an inch or so of alcohol above the herb mixture.

4. Seal the jar tightly and give it a good shake to mix the ingredients.

5. Store the jar in a cool, dark place, and shake it daily for about 4-6 weeks.

6. After the steeping period, strain the tincture through a muslin cloth or a fine mesh strainer to remove the herb solids.

7. Transfer the liquid into a glass dropper bottle.

8. Take 1-2 dropperfuls (about 30-60 drops) of the tincture in a small amount of water as needed for allergies.

<u>**CALENDULA AND CHAMOMILE:**</u>

INGREDIENTS:

- 2 parts dried Calendula flowers
- 1 part dried Chamomile flowers
- 80-100 proof alcohol

INSTRUCTIONS:

1. Combine the dried Calendula flowers and dried Chamomile flowers in a glass jar with a tight-fitting lid.
2. Fill the jar halfway with the herb mixture.
3. Pour enough alcohol over the herbs to fully cover them with an inch or so of alcohol above the herb mixture.
4. Seal the jar tightly and give it a good shake to mix the ingredients.
5. Store the jar in a cool, dark place, and shake it daily for about 4-6 weeks.
6. After the steeping period, strain the tincture through a muslin cloth or a fine mesh strainer to remove the herb solids.
7. Transfer the liquid into a glass dropper bottle.
8. Take 1-2 dropperfuls (about 30-60 drops) of the tincture in a small amount of water as needed for allergies.

**Remember to consult with a healthcare professional before using these tinctures, especially if you have any underlying health conditions, are taking medications, or are pregnant or breastfeeding.**

DIGESTIVE DISORDERS

GINGER AND PEPPERMINT:

INGREDIENTS:

- 2 parts dried Ginger root

- 1 part dried Peppermint leaf

- 80-100 proof alcohol

INSTRUCTIONS:

1. Combine the dried Ginger root and dried Peppermint leaf in a glass jar with a tight-fitting lid.

2. Fill the jar halfway with the herb mixture.

3. Pour enough alcohol over the herbs to fully cover them with an inch or so of alcohol above the herb mixture.

4. Seal the jar tightly and give it a good shake to mix the ingredients.

5. Store the jar in a cool, dark place, and shake it daily for about 4-6 weeks.

6. After the steeping period, strain the tincture through a muslin cloth or a fine mesh strainer to remove the herb solids.

7. Transfer the liquid into a glass dropper bottle.

8. Take 1-2 dropperfuls (about 30-60 drops) of the tincture in a small amount of water as needed for digestive disorders.

<u>**FENNEL AND CHAMOMILE:**</u>

INGREDIENTS:

- 2 parts dried Fennel seeds
- 1 part dried Chamomile flowers
- 80-100 proof alcohol

INSTRUCTIONS:

1. Combine the dried Fennel seeds and dried Chamomile flowers in a glass jar with a tight-fitting lid.
2. Fill the jar halfway with the herb mixture.
3. Pour enough alcohol over the herbs to fully cover them with an inch or so of alcohol above the herb mixture.
4. Seal the jar tightly and give it a good shake to mix the ingredients.
5. Store the jar in a cool, dark place, and shake it daily for about 4-6 weeks.
6. After the steeping period, strain the tincture through a muslin cloth or a fine mesh strainer to remove the herb solids.
7. Transfer the liquid into a glass dropper bottle.
8. Take 1-2 dropperfuls (about 30-60 drops) of the tincture in a small amount of water as needed for digestive disorders.

<u>Remember to consult with a healthcare professional before using these tinctures, especially if you have any underlying health conditions, are taking medications, or are pregnant or breastfeeding.</u>

ST. JOHN'S WORT AND LEMON BALM:

INGREDIENTS:

- 2 parts dried St. John's Wort flowers and leaves

- 1 part dried Lemon Balm leaves

- 80-100 proof alcohol

INSTRUCTIONS:

1. Combine the dried St. John's Wort and Lemon Balm in a glass jar with a tight-fitting lid.

2. Fill the jar halfway with the herb mixture.

3. Pour enough alcohol over the herbs to fully cover them with an inch or so of alcohol above the herb mixture.

4. Seal the jar tightly and give it a good shake to mix the ingredients.

5. Store the jar in a cool, dark place, and shake it daily for about 4-6 weeks.

6. After the steeping period, strain the tincture through a muslin cloth or a fine mesh strainer to remove the herb solids.

7. Transfer the liquid into a glass dropper bottle.

8. Take 1-2 dropperfuls (about 30-60 drops) of the tincture in a small amount of water up to three times daily to support emotional well-being.

PASSIONFLOWER AND SKULLCAP:

INGREDIENTS:

- 2 parts dried Passionflower aerial parts
- 1 part dried Skullcap aerial parts
- 80-100 proof alcohol

INSTRUCTIONS:

1. Combine the dried Passionflower and Skullcap in a glass jar with a tight-fitting lid.
2. Fill the jar halfway with the herb mixture.
3. Pour enough alcohol over the herbs to fully cover them with an inch or so of alcohol above the herb mixture.
4. Seal the jar tightly and give it a good shake to mix the ingredients.
5. Store the jar in a cool, dark place, and shake it daily for about 4-6 weeks.
6. After the steeping period, strain the tincture through a muslin cloth or a fine mesh strainer to remove the herb solids.
7. Transfer the liquid into a glass dropper bottle.
8. Take 1-2 dropperfuls (about 30-60 drops) of the tincture in a small amount of water up to three times daily to support emotional well-being.

Please note that herbal remedies may not be suitable for everyone, and it's essential to consult with a healthcare professional before using these tinctures, especially if you have any underlying health conditions, are taking medications, or are pregnant or breastfeeding.

CHAMOMILE AND LAVENDER:

INGREDIENTS:

- 2 parts dried Chamomile flowers

- 1 part dried Lavender flowers

- 80-100 proof alcohol

INSTRUCTIONS:

1. Combine the dried Chamomile and Lavender in a glass jar with a tight-fitting lid.

2. Fill the jar halfway with the herb mixture.

3. Pour enough alcohol over the herbs to fully cover them with an inch or so of alcohol above the herb mixture.

4. Seal the jar tightly and give it a good shake to mix the ingredients.

5. Store the jar in a cool, dark place, and shake it daily for about 4-6 weeks.

6. After the steeping period, strain the tincture through a muslin cloth or a fine mesh strainer to remove the herb solids.

7. Transfer the liquid into a glass dropper bottle.

8. Take 1-2 dropperfuls (about 30-60 drops) of the tincture in a small amount of water up to three times daily to help promote a sense of calm and relaxation.

<u>**LEMON BALM AND PASSIONFLOWER:**</u>

INGREDIENTS:

- 2 parts dried Lemon Balm leaves
- 1 part dried Passionflower aerial parts
- 80-100 proof alcohol

INSTRUCTIONS:

1. Combine the dried Lemon Balm and Passionflower in a glass jar with a tight-fitting lid.
2. Fill the jar halfway with the herb mixture.
3. Pour enough alcohol over the herbs to fully cover them with an inch or so of alcohol above the herb mixture.
4. Seal the jar tightly and give it a good shake to mix the ingredients.
5. Store the jar in a cool, dark place, and shake it daily for about 4-6 weeks.
6. After the steeping period, strain the tincture through a muslin cloth or a fine mesh strainer to remove the herb solids.
7. Transfer the liquid into a glass dropper bottle.
8. Take 1-2 dropperfuls (about 30-60 drops) of the tincture in a small amount of water up to three times daily to help promote relaxation and ease anxiety.

**It's important to consult with a healthcare professional before using these tinctures if you have any underlying health conditions, are taking medications, or are pregnant or breastfeeding. They can provide guidance on the appropriate dosage and how these herbs may interact with any existing treatments you may be undergoing.**

MOOD DISORDERS

While herbal tinctures may offer potential benefits for certain health conditions, it is important to note that bipolar disorder is a serious mental health condition that requires professional medical attention. Herbal remedies should not be used as a substitute for prescribed medications, therapy, or other treatments for bipolar disorder.

That said, some herbs may have a calming effect and be generally supportive for overall well-being. However, their specific impact on bipolar disorder symptoms can vary from person to person. It is crucial to consult with a healthcare professional or a qualified herbalist who can provide guidance tailored to your specific needs and circumstances. They can help you determine if herbal remedies might be safe and appropriate for you, while still maintaining your prescribed treatment plan.

I can suggest some combinations of herbs that are commonly used in alcohol-based tinctures for mood disorders:

ST. JOHN'S WORT, LEMON BALM, AND PASSIONFLOWER:

This combination may help promote relaxation, uplift mood, and reduce anxiety.

ASHWAGANDHA, RHODIOLA ROSEA, AND SKULLCAP:

These adaptogenic herbs may help reduce stress, support a balanced mood, and promote relaxation.

LEMON BALM, LAVENDER, AND CHAMOMILE:

This combination of calming herbs can help alleviate anxiety, induce relaxation, and improve sleep quality.

HOLY BASIL, ST. JOHN'S WORT, AND VALERIAN:

This blend may help support a positive mood, reduce stress and anxiety, and promote restful sleep.

GINKGO BILOBA, GOTU KOLA, AND SIBERIAN GINSENG:

This combination can enhance cognitive function, improve mental clarity, and support mood stability.

Please keep in mind that these are general suggestions, and it is important to consult with a qualified herbalist or healthcare professional for personalized advice based on your specific needs and health condition. They can provide detailed guidance on preparation methods, dosing, and potential interactions or contraindications.

*Creating alcohol-based tinctures for ADHD requires a careful selection of herbs and proper dosage. **Here are some herb combinations that are commonly used in tincture recipes for ADHD:***

LEMON BALM (MELISSA OFFICINALIS) AND SKULLCAP (SCUTELLARIA LATERIFLORA):

Lemon balm has calming properties, while skullcap helps with focus and concentration.

GINKGO BILOBA (GINKGO BILOBA) AND GOTU KOLA (CENTELLA ASIATICA):

Ginkgo biloba may enhance cognitive function, while gotu kola is believed to support mental clarity and brain health.

CHAMOMILE (MATRICARIA CHAMOMILLA) AND PASSIONFLOWER (PASSIFLORA INCARNATA):

Chamomile has relaxing effects, while passionflower helps reduce restlessness.

VALERIAN (VALERIANA OFFICINALIS) AND CALIFORNIA POPPY (ESCHSCHOLZIA CALIFORNICA):

Valerian is known for its sedative properties, while California poppy may help reduce hyperactivity.

LAVENDER (LAVANDULA ANGUSTIFOLIA) AND LEMON VERBENA (ALOYSIA CITRODORA):

Lavender promotes relaxation, and lemon verbena may support focus and reduce anxiety.

Remember, it's crucial to consult with a qualified herbalist or healthcare professional to get personalized advice and guidance on the correct dosages and potential herb interactions. They can help customize a tincture recipe based on your specific needs and preferences.

SUBSTANCE ABUSE DISORDERS

Creating alcohol-based tinctures for substance abuse disorders requires careful consideration and guidance from healthcare professionals. **However, here are some herbs that are often used in tinctures for supporting substance abuse recovery:**

MILK THISTLE (SILYBUM MARIANUM):

Known for its liver-protective properties, milk thistle may help support the liver during detoxification processes.

ST. JOHN'S WORT (HYPERICUM PERFORATUM):

St. John's Wort is believed to have mood-stabilizing effects and may help ease withdrawal symptoms and support mental health.

KUDZU ROOT (PUERARIA LOBATA):

Kudzu root is commonly used in traditional Chinese medicine to reduce alcohol cravings and support sobriety.

PASSIONFLOWER (PASSIFLORA INCARNATA):

Passionflower may have calming properties and help reduce anxiety and restlessness associated with substance withdrawal.

VALERIAN (VALERIANA OFFICINALIS):

Valerian has sedative effects and may support relaxation and restful sleep, which can be beneficial during substance abuse recovery.

Please note that these suggestions are not a substitute for professional advice. I strongly recommend consulting with a qualified healthcare provider or herbalist who specializes in substance abuse recovery to get personalized guidance and

In conclusion, harnessing the power of nature for wellness and incorporating the use of herbal tinctures can have profound positive impacts on our overall health and well-being. Throughout history, humans have relied on the healing properties of plants and herbs to treat various ailments and promote vitality.

Today, with the advancements in herbal medicine and the availability of high-quality herbal tinctures, we have a wide range of natural remedies at our disposal. Herbal tinctures are concentrated extracts of plant material infused in alcohol or other solvents, preserving the beneficial compounds and making them easily accessible for therapeutic use.

One of the key advantages of herbal tinctures is their versatility. They can be custom made to address specific health concerns, tailored to individual needs and preferences. Whether it's managing stress, supporting digestion, boosting immunity, or enhancing sleep quality, there is likely an herbal tincture that can provide the desired effects.

Furthermore, the use of herbal tinctures allows for greater control over dosage. By starting low and gradually increasing, one can find the optimal dosage for maximum therapeutic benefit. This personalized approach ensures that the body receives the right amount of active constituents while minimizing potential side effects.

Harnessing the power of nature for wellness also encourages a holistic approach to our health. By embracing the wisdom of nature and incorporating herbal tinctures into our daily routines, we are reminded of the interconnectedness between our bodies, minds, and the natural world. This mindful approach can lead to a deeper sense of well-being and harmony.

However, it is essential to always seek guidance from healthcare professionals or herbalists when incorporating herbal tinctures into our wellness regimens. They can provide expert advice on dosage, possible interactions with medications, and help tailor treatment plans to individual needs.

In conclusion, by harnessing the power of nature through the use of herbal tinctures, we can tap into the vast healing potential of plants and herbs. Whether used as supportive remedies or as part of a comprehensive wellness routine, herbal tinctures offer a natural and effective means to enhance our overall health, vitality, and connection with the world around us.

GLOSSARY

TINCTURE:
A concentrated liquid extract made from herbs using alcohol or a solvent.

ALCOHOL-BASED TINCTURE:
A tincture made by steeping herbs in alcohol to extract their active compounds.

SOLVENT:
A substance used to extract the active compounds from herbs. Alcohol is a commonly used solvent in tincture making.

HERBALISM:
The practice of using plants and their extracts for therapeutic purposes.

EXTRACTION:
The process of obtaining the active compounds from herbs for use in tincture making.

MACERATION:
The process of soaking herbs in a solvent to extract their active compounds.

MENSTRUUM:
The liquid used as a solvent for extracting and preserving the active compounds in a tincture.

HERBAL REMEDY:
A natural treatment made from plants and their extracts to address specific health conditions.

HERBAL CONSTITUENTS:
The bioactive compounds found in plants that provide therapeutic benefits.

CONSTITUENT EXTRACTION:
The process of extracting specific compounds from herbs to enhance their medicinal properties.

HERBAL PREPARATION:
A product made from herbs, such as tinctures, teas, capsules, or salves.

HERBAL FOLKLORE:
Traditional beliefs and practices related to the use of herbs for healing purposes.

HERBAL SAFETY:
The practice of ensuring the proper dosage and appropriate use of herbal products to avoid adverse effects.

HERBAL PHARMACOLOGY:
The study of how herbs interact with the body and produce therapeutic effects.

HERBAL DOSAGE:
The recommended amount of herbal preparation to be taken for a specific condition or desired effect.

HERBAL SYNERGIES:
The combined effects of multiple herbs when used together in a tincture or herbal formula.

HERBAL MONOGRAPHS:
Detailed profiles or summaries of individual herbs, including their properties, uses, and potential interactions.

HERB-DRUG INTERACTIONS:
The effects and potential contraindications when herbs are used in conjunction with pharmaceutical drugs.

HERBAL SUSTAINABILITY:
The practice of using herbs in a way that ensures their long-term availability and minimizes environmental impact.

QUALITY CONTROL:
Measures taken to ensure the purity, potency, and consistency
of herbal tinctures through standardized production processes.

CITED SOURCES & RESOURCES

Balch, P. A., & Balch, J. F. (2012). Prescription for Herbal Healing: An Easy-to-Use A-Z Reference to Hundreds of Common Disorders and Their Herbal Remedies. Penguin.

Bone, K., & Mills, S. (2013). Principles and Practice of Phytotherapy: Modern Herbal Medicine. Churchill Livingstone.

Gladstar, R. (2001). Herbal Healing for Women: Simple Home Remedies for Women of All Ages. Simon and Schuster.

Hoffman, D. (2003). Medical Herbalism: The Science and Practice of Herbal Medicine. Healing Arts Press.

Mills, S., & Bone, K. (2005). The Essential Guide to Herbal Safety. Elsevier Health Sciences.

Moore, M. (1996). Medicinal Plants of the Mountain West. Museum of New Mexico Press.

Tierra, M. (2003). The Way of Herbs. Pocket Books.

Weed, S. S. (1989). Wise Woman Herbal for the Childbearing Year. Ash Tree Publishing.

Winston, D., & Maimes, S. (2007). Adaptogens: Herbs for Strength, Stamina, and Stress Relief. Inner Traditions/Bear & Co.

Wood, M. (2008). The Earthwise Herbal: A Complete Guide to Old World Medicinal Plants. North Atlantic Books.

Yance, D. R. (2013). Adaptogens in Medical Herbalism: Elite Herbs and Natural Compounds for Mastering Stress, Aging, and Chronic Disease. Healing Arts Press.

World Health Organization. (2002). WHO Monographs on Selected Medicinal Plants. Volume 2. World Health Organization.

Grieve, M. (1971). A Modern Herbal. Dover Publications.

Mabey, R. (1997). New Age Herbalist: How to Use Herbs for Healing, Nutrition, Body Care, and Relaxation. Simon and Schuster.

Chevallier, A. (2016). Encyclopedia of Herbal Medicine. DK.

Bove, M. (2009). An Encyclopedia of Natural Healing for Children and Infants. Keats Publishing.

Hoffmann, D. (1990). The New Holistic Herbal. Element Books.

Duke, J. A., & Foster, S. (2003). Peterson Field Guide to Medicinal Plants and Herbs of Eastern and Central North America. Houghton Mifflin Harcourt.

Fritchey, P. (2004). Practical Herbalism: Ordinary Plants with Extraordinary Powers. First Facts Books.

Holmes, P. (2007). The Energetics of Western Herbs: A Materia Medica Integrating Western and Chinese Herbal Therapeutics. Snow Lotus Press.

CREATE YOUR OWN TINCTURE
TINCTURE NAME & SPECIFIC AILMENT OR CONCERN:

INGREDIENTS:

1. -
2. -
3. -
4. -
5. -

PREPARATION:

Combine equal parts of each herb (e.g., 1 ounce or 30 grams each) in a glass jar. Cover them with vodka or another high-proof alcohol, ensuring all the herbs are submerged. Seal the jar tightly.

Shake the jar daily for 4-6 weeks to allow the alcohol to extract the medicinal compounds.

STORAGE:

Store the jar in a cool, dark place. After 4-6 weeks, strain the tincture using cheesecloth or a fine-mesh strainer, and transfer the liquid into amber glass dropper bottles for easy use. This tincture can be stored for up to 5 years.

ADDITIONAL INFORMATION:

Remember to label your tinctures with the ingredients and date of preparation. Start with small doses (e.g., a dropperful) and gradually increase if needed.

CREATE YOUR OWN TINCTURE
TINCTURE NAME & SPECIFIC AILMENT OR CONCERN:

**INGREDIENTS:**
1. -
2. -
3. -
4. -
5. -

PREPARATION:

Combine equal parts of each herb (e.g., 1 ounce or 30 grams each) in a glass jar. Cover them with vodka or another high-proof alcohol, ensuring all the herbs are submerged. Seal the jar tightly.

Shake the jar daily for 4-6 weeks to allow the alcohol to extract the medicinal compounds.

STORAGE:

Store the jar in a cool, dark place. After 4-6 weeks, strain the tincture using cheesecloth or a fine-mesh strainer, and transfer the liquid into amber glass dropper bottles for easy use. This tincture can be stored for up to 5 years.

ADDITIONAL INFORMATION:

**Remember to label your tinctures with the ingredients and date of preparation. Start with small doses (e.g., a dropperful) and gradually increase if needed.**

TINCTURE NAME & SPECIFIC AILMENT OR CONCERN:

INGREDIENTS:

1. -
2. -
3. -
4. -
5. -

PREPARATION:

Combine equal parts of each herb (e.g., 1 ounce or 30 grams each) in a glass jar. Cover them with vodka or another high-proof alcohol, ensuring all the herbs are submerged. Seal the jar tightly.

Shake the jar daily for 4-6 weeks to allow the alcohol to extract the medicinal compounds.

STORAGE:

Store the jar in a cool, dark place. After 4-6 weeks, strain the tincture using cheesecloth or a fine-mesh strainer, and transfer the liquid into amber glass dropper bottles for easy use. This tincture can be stored for up to 5 years.

ADDITIONAL INFORMATION:

Remember to label your tinctures with the ingredients and date of preparation. Start with small doses (e.g., a dropperful) and gradually increase if needed.

CREATE YOUR OWN TINCTURE
TINCTURE NAME & SPECIFIC AILMENT OR CONCERN:

INGREDIENTS:
1. -
2. -
3. -
4. -
5. -

PREPARATION:

Combine equal parts of each herb (e.g., 1 ounce or 30 grams each) in a glass jar. Cover them with vodka or another high-proof alcohol, ensuring all the herbs are submerged. Seal the jar tightly.

Shake the jar daily for 4-6 weeks to allow the alcohol to extract the medicinal compounds.

STORAGE:

Store the jar in a cool, dark place. After 4-6 weeks, strain the tincture using cheesecloth or a fine-mesh strainer, and transfer the liquid into amber glass dropper bottles for easy use. This tincture can be stored for up to 5 years.

ADDITIONAL INFORMATION:

**Remember to label your tinctures with the ingredients and date of preparation. Start with small doses (e.g., a dropperful) and gradually increase if needed.**

CREATE YOUR OWN TINCTURE

TINCTURE NAME & SPECIFIC AILMENT OR CONCERN:

INGREDIENTS:

1. -
2. -
3. -
4. -
5. -

PREPARATION:

Combine equal parts of each herb (e.g., 1 ounce or 30 grams each) in a glass jar. Cover them with vodka or another high-proof alcohol, ensuring all the herbs are submerged. Seal the jar tightly.

Shake the jar daily for 4-6 weeks to allow the alcohol to extract the medicinal compounds.

STORAGE:

Store the jar in a cool, dark place. After 4-6 weeks, strain the tincture using cheesecloth or a fine-mesh strainer, and transfer the liquid into amber glass dropper bottles for easy use. This tincture can be stored for up to 5 years.

ADDITIONAL INFORMATION:

Remember to label your tinctures with the ingredients and date of preparation. Start with small doses (e.g., a dropperful) and gradually increase if needed.

CREATE YOUR OWN TINCTURE
TINCTURE NAME & SPECIFIC AILMENT OR CONCERN:

<u>*INGREDIENTS:*</u>
1. -
2. -
3. -
4. -
5. -

<u>*PREPARATION:*</u>

Combine equal parts of each herb (e.g., 1 ounce or 30 grams each) in a glass jar. Cover them with vodka or another high-proof alcohol, ensuring all the herbs are submerged. Seal the jar tightly.

Shake the jar daily for 4-6 weeks to allow the alcohol to extract the medicinal compounds.

<u>*STORAGE:*</u>

Store the jar in a cool, dark place. After 4-6 weeks, strain the tincture using cheesecloth or a fine-mesh strainer, and transfer the liquid into amber glass dropper bottles for easy use. This tincture can be stored for up to 5 years.

<u>*ADDITIONAL INFORMATION:*</u>

<u>*Remember to label your tinctures with the ingredients and date of preparation. Start with small doses (e.g., a dropperful) and gradually increase if needed.*</u>

TINCTURE NAME & SPECIFIC AILMENT OR CONCERN:

INGREDIENTS:

1. -
2. -
3. -
4. -
5. -

PREPARATION:

Combine equal parts of each herb (e.g., 1 ounce or 30 grams each) in a glass jar. Cover them with vodka or another high-proof alcohol, ensuring all the herbs are submerged. Seal the jar tightly.

Shake the jar daily for 4-6 weeks to allow the alcohol to extract the medicinal compounds.

STORAGE:

Store the jar in a cool, dark place. After 4-6 weeks, strain the tincture using cheesecloth or a fine-mesh strainer, and transfer the liquid into amber glass dropper bottles for easy use. This tincture can be stored for up to 5 years.

ADDITIONAL INFORMATION:

Remember to label your tinctures with the ingredients and date of preparation. Start with small doses (e.g., a dropperful) and gradually increase if needed.

CREATE YOUR OWN TINCTURE
TINCTURE NAME & SPECIFIC AILMENT OR CONCERN:

INGREDIENTS:

1. -
2. -
3. -
4. -
5. -

PREPARATION:

Combine equal parts of each herb (e.g., 1 ounce or 30 grams each) in a glass jar. Cover them with vodka or another high-proof alcohol, ensuring all the herbs are submerged. Seal the jar tightly.

Shake the jar daily for 4-6 weeks to allow the alcohol to extract the medicinal compounds.

STORAGE:

Store the jar in a cool, dark place. After 4-6 weeks, strain the tincture using cheesecloth or a fine-mesh strainer, and transfer the liquid into amber glass dropper bottles for easy use. This tincture can be stored for up to 5 years.

ADDITIONAL INFORMATION:

Remember to label your tinctures with the ingredients and date of preparation. Start with small doses (e.g., a dropperful) and gradually increase if needed.

CREATE YOUR OWN TINCTURE
TINCTURE NAME & SPECIFIC AILMENT OR CONCERN:

INGREDIENTS:
1. -
2. -
3. -
4. -
5. -

PREPARATION:

Combine equal parts of each herb (e.g., 1 ounce or 30 grams each) in a glass jar. Cover them with vodka or another high-proof alcohol, ensuring all the herbs are submerged. Seal the jar tightly.

Shake the jar daily for 4-6 weeks to allow the alcohol to extract the medicinal compounds.

STORAGE:

Store the jar in a cool, dark place. After 4-6 weeks, strain the tincture using cheesecloth or a fine-mesh strainer, and transfer the liquid into amber glass dropper bottles for easy use. This tincture can be stored for up to 5 years.

ADDITIONAL INFORMATION:

Remember to label your tinctures with the ingredients and date of preparation. Start with small doses (e.g., a dropperful) and gradually increase if needed.

CREATE YOUR OWN TINCTURE
TINCTURE NAME & SPECIFIC AILMENT OR CONCERN:

INGREDIENTS:

1. -
2. -
3. -
4. -
5. -

PREPARATION:

Combine equal parts of each herb (e.g., 1 ounce or 30 grams each) in a glass jar. Cover them with vodka or another high-proof alcohol, ensuring all the herbs are submerged. Seal the jar tightly.

Shake the jar daily for 4-6 weeks to allow the alcohol to extract the medicinal compounds.

STORAGE:

Store the jar in a cool, dark place. After 4-6 weeks, strain the tincture using cheesecloth or a fine-mesh strainer, and transfer the liquid into amber glass dropper bottles for easy use. This tincture can be stored for up to 5 years.

ADDITIONAL INFORMATION:

Remember to label your tinctures with the ingredients and date of preparation. Start with small doses (e.g., a dropperful) and gradually increase if needed.

TINCTURE NAME & SPECIFIC AILMENT OR CONCERN:

INGREDIENTS:

1. -
2. -
3. -
4. -
5. -

PREPARATION:

Combine equal parts of each herb (e.g., 1 ounce or 30 grams each) in a glass jar. Cover them with vodka or another high-proof alcohol, ensuring all the herbs are submerged. Seal the jar tightly.

Shake the jar daily for 4-6 weeks to allow the alcohol to extract the medicinal compounds.

STORAGE:

Store the jar in a cool, dark place. After 4-6 weeks, strain the tincture using cheesecloth or a fine-mesh strainer, and transfer the liquid into amber glass dropper bottles for easy use. This tincture can be stored for up to 5 years.

ADDITIONAL INFORMATION:

Remember to label your tinctures with the ingredients and date of preparation. Start with small doses (e.g., a dropperful) and gradually increase if needed.

CREATE YOUR OWN TINCTURE
TINCTURE NAME & SPECIFIC AILMENT OR CONCERN:

INGREDIENTS:

1. -
2. -
3. -
4. -
5. -

PREPARATION:

Combine equal parts of each herb (e.g., 1 ounce or 30 grams each) in a glass jar. Cover them with vodka or another high-proof alcohol, ensuring all the herbs are submerged. Seal the jar tightly.

Shake the jar daily for 4-6 weeks to allow the alcohol to extract the medicinal compounds.

STORAGE:

Store the jar in a cool, dark place. After 4-6 weeks, strain the tincture using cheesecloth or a fine-mesh strainer, and transfer the liquid into amber glass dropper bottles for easy use. This tincture can be stored for up to 5 years.

ADDITIONAL INFORMATION:

Remember to label your tinctures with the ingredients and date of preparation. Start with small doses (e.g., a dropperful) and gradually increase if needed.

CREATE YOUR OWN TINCTURE
TINCTURE NAME & SPECIFIC AILMENT OR CONCERN:

<u>*INGREDIENTS:*</u>
1. -
2. -
3. -
4. -
5. -

PREPARATION:

Combine equal parts of each herb (e.g., 1 ounce or 30 grams each) in a glass jar. Cover them with vodka or another high-proof alcohol, ensuring all the herbs are submerged. Seal the jar tightly.

Shake the jar daily for 4-6 weeks to allow the alcohol to extract the medicinal compounds.

STORAGE:

Store the jar in a cool, dark place. After 4-6 weeks, strain the tincture using cheesecloth or a fine-mesh strainer, and transfer the liquid into amber glass dropper bottles for easy use. This tincture can be stored for up to 5 years.

<u>ADDITIONAL INFORMATION:</u>

<u>***Remember to label your tinctures with the ingredients and date of preparation. Start with small doses (e.g., a dropperful) and gradually increase if needed.***</u>

CREATE YOUR OWN TINCTURE
TINCTURE NAME & SPECIFIC AILMENT OR CONCERN:

INGREDIENTS:
1. -
2. -
3. -
4. -
5. -

PREPARATION:

Combine equal parts of each herb (e.g., 1 ounce or 30 grams each) in a glass jar. Cover them with vodka or another high-proof alcohol, ensuring all the herbs are submerged. Seal the jar tightly.

Shake the jar daily for 4-6 weeks to allow the alcohol to extract the medicinal compounds.

STORAGE:

Store the jar in a cool, dark place. After 4-6 weeks, strain the tincture using cheesecloth or a fine-mesh strainer, and transfer the liquid into amber glass dropper bottles for easy use. This tincture can be stored for up to 5 years.

ADDITIONAL INFORMATION:

Remember to label your tinctures with the ingredients and date of preparation. Start with small doses (e.g., a dropperful) and gradually increase if needed.

CREATE YOUR OWN TINCTURE
TINCTURE NAME & SPECIFIC AILMENT OR CONCERN:

INGREDIENTS:

1. -
2. -
3. -
4. -
5. -

PREPARATION:

Combine equal parts of each herb (e.g., 1 ounce or 30 grams each) in a glass jar. Cover them with vodka or another high-proof alcohol, ensuring all the herbs are submerged. Seal the jar tightly.

Shake the jar daily for 4-6 weeks to allow the alcohol to extract the medicinal compounds.

STORAGE:

Store the jar in a cool, dark place. After 4-6 weeks, strain the tincture using cheesecloth or a fine-mesh strainer, and transfer the liquid into amber glass dropper bottles for easy use. This tincture can be stored for up to 5 years.

ADDITIONAL INFORMATION:

Remember to label your tinctures with the ingredients and date of preparation. Start with small doses (e.g., a dropperful) and gradually increase if needed.

CREATE YOUR OWN TINCTURE
TINCTURE NAME & SPECIFIC AILMENT OR CONCERN:

INGREDIENTS:
1. -
2. -
3. -
4. -
5. -

PREPARATION:

Combine equal parts of each herb (e.g., 1 ounce or 30 grams each) in a glass jar. Cover them with vodka or another high-proof alcohol, ensuring all the herbs are submerged. Seal the jar tightly.

Shake the jar daily for 4-6 weeks to allow the alcohol to extract the medicinal compounds.

STORAGE:

Store the jar in a cool, dark place. After 4-6 weeks, strain the tincture using cheesecloth or a fine-mesh strainer, and transfer the liquid into amber glass dropper bottles for easy use. This tincture can be stored for up to 5 years.

ADDITIONAL INFORMATION:

**Remember to label your tinctures with the ingredients and date of preparation. Start with small doses (e.g., a dropperful) and gradually increase if needed.**

CREATE YOUR OWN TINCTURE
TINCTURE NAME & SPECIFIC AILMENT OR CONCERN:

INGREDIENTS:

1. -
2. -
3. -
4. -
5. -

PREPARATION:

Combine equal parts of each herb (e.g., 1 ounce or 30 grams each) in a glass jar. Cover them with vodka or another high-proof alcohol, ensuring all the herbs are submerged. Seal the jar tightly.

Shake the jar daily for 4-6 weeks to allow the alcohol to extract the medicinal compounds.

STORAGE:

Store the jar in a cool, dark place. After 4-6 weeks, strain the tincture using cheesecloth or a fine-mesh strainer, and transfer the liquid into amber glass dropper bottles for easy use. This tincture can be stored for up to 5 years.

ADDITIONAL INFORMATION:

Remember to label your tinctures with the ingredients and date of preparation. Start with small doses (e.g., a dropperful) and gradually increase if needed.

CREATE YOUR OWN TINCTURE
TINCTURE NAME & SPECIFIC AILMENT OR CONCERN:

INGREDIENTS:

1. -
2. -
3. -
4. -
5. -

PREPARATION:

Combine equal parts of each herb (e.g., 1 ounce or 30 grams each) in a glass jar. Cover them with vodka or another high-proof alcohol, ensuring all the herbs are submerged. Seal the jar tightly.

Shake the jar daily for 4-6 weeks to allow the alcohol to extract the medicinal compounds.

STORAGE:

Store the jar in a cool, dark place. After 4-6 weeks, strain the tincture using cheesecloth or a fine-mesh strainer, and transfer the liquid into amber glass dropper bottles for easy use. This tincture can be stored for up to 5 years.

ADDITIONAL INFORMATION:

**Remember to label your tinctures with the ingredients and date of preparation. Start with small doses (e.g., a dropperful) and gradually increase if needed.**

CREATE YOUR OWN TINCTURE
TINCTURE NAME & SPECIFIC AILMENT OR CONCERN:

**INGREDIENTS:**
1. -
2. -
3. -
4. -
5. -

**PREPARATION:**

Combine equal parts of each herb (e.g., 1 ounce or 30 grams each) in a glass jar. Cover them with vodka or another high-proof alcohol, ensuring all the herbs are submerged. Seal the jar tightly.

Shake the jar daily for 4-6 weeks to allow the alcohol to extract the medicinal compounds.

**STORAGE:**

Store the jar in a cool, dark place. After 4-6 weeks, strain the tincture using cheesecloth or a fine-mesh strainer, and transfer the liquid into amber glass dropper bottles for easy use. This tincture can be stored for up to 5 years.

ADDITIONAL INFORMATION:

Remember to label your tinctures with the ingredients and date of preparation. Start with small doses (e.g., a dropperful) and gradually increase if needed

CREATE YOUR OWN TINCTURE
TINCTURE NAME & SPECIFIC AILMENT OR CONCERN:

INGREDIENTS:
1.   -
2.   -
3.   -
4.   -
5.   -

PREPARATION:

Combine equal parts of each herb (e.g., 1 ounce or 30 grams each) in a glass jar. Cover them with vodka or another high-proof alcohol, ensuring all the herbs are submerged. Seal the jar tightly.

Shake the jar daily for 4-6 weeks to allow the alcohol to extract the medicinal compounds.

STORAGE:

Store the jar in a cool, dark place. After 4-6 weeks, strain the tincture using cheesecloth or a fine-mesh strainer, and transfer the liquid into amber glass dropper bottles for easy use. This tincture can be stored for up to 5 years.

ADDITIONAL INFORMATION:

Remember to label your tinctures with the ingredients and date of preparation. Start with small doses (e.g., a dropperful) and gradually increase if needed.

CREATE YOUR OWN TINCTURE
TINCTURE NAME & SPECIFIC AILMENT OR CONCERN:

INGREDIENTS:

1. -
2. -
3. -
4. -
5. -

PREPARATION:

Combine equal parts of each herb (e.g., 1 ounce or 30 grams each) in a glass jar. Cover them with vodka or another high-proof alcohol, ensuring all the herbs are submerged. Seal the jar tightly.

Shake the jar daily for 4-6 weeks to allow the alcohol to extract the medicinal compounds.

STORAGE:

Store the jar in a cool, dark place. After 4-6 weeks, strain the tincture using cheesecloth or a fine-mesh strainer, and transfer the liquid into amber glass dropper bottles for easy use. This tincture can be stored for up to 5 years.

ADDITIONAL INFORMATION:

**Remember to label your tinctures with the ingredients and date of preparation. Start with small doses (e.g., a dropperful) and gradually increase if needed.**

CREATE YOUR OWN TINCTURE

TINCTURE NAME & SPECIFIC AILMENT OR CONCERN:

INGREDIENTS:

1. -
2. -
3. -
4. -
5. -

PREPARATION:

Combine equal parts of each herb (e.g., 1 ounce or 30 grams each) in a glass jar. Cover them with vodka or another high-proof alcohol, ensuring all the herbs are submerged. Seal the jar tightly.

Shake the jar daily for 4-6 weeks to allow the alcohol to extract the medicinal compounds.

STORAGE:

Store the jar in a cool, dark place. After 4-6 weeks, strain the tincture using cheesecloth or a fine-mesh strainer, and transfer the liquid into amber glass dropper bottles for easy use. This tincture can be stored for up to 5 years.

ADDITIONAL INFORMATION:

Remember to label your tinctures with the ingredients and date of preparation. Start with small doses (e.g., a dropperful) and gradually increase if needed.

CREATE YOUR OWN TINCTURE
TINCTURE NAME & SPECIFIC AILMENT OR CONCERN:

INGREDIENTS:

1. -
2. -
3. -
4. -
5. -

PREPARATION:

Combine equal parts of each herb (e.g., 1 ounce or 30 grams each) in a glass jar. Cover them with vodka or another high-proof alcohol, ensuring all the herbs are submerged. Seal the jar tightly.

Shake the jar daily for 4-6 weeks to allow the alcohol to extract the medicinal compounds.

STORAGE:

Store the jar in a cool, dark place. After 4-6 weeks, strain the tincture using cheesecloth or a fine-mesh strainer, and transfer the liquid into amber glass dropper bottles for easy use. This tincture can be stored for up to 5 years.

ADDITIONAL INFORMATION:

Remember to label your tinctures with the ingredients and date of preparation. Start with small doses (e.g., a dropperful) and gradually increase if needed.

CREATE YOUR OWN TINCTURE
TINCTURE NAME & SPECIFIC AILMENT OR CONCERN:

INGREDIENTS:
1. -
2. -
3. -
4. -
5. -

PREPARATION:

Combine equal parts of each herb (e.g., 1 ounce or 30 grams each) in a glass jar. Cover them with vodka or another high-proof alcohol, ensuring all the herbs are submerged. Seal the jar tightly.

Shake the jar daily for 4-6 weeks to allow the alcohol to extract the medicinal compounds.

STORAGE:

Store the jar in a cool, dark place. After 4-6 weeks, strain the tincture using cheesecloth or a fine-mesh strainer, and transfer the liquid into amber glass dropper bottles for easy use. This tincture can be stored for up to 5 years.

ADDITIONAL INFORMATION:

Remember to label your tinctures with the ingredients and date of preparation. Start with small doses (e.g., a dropperful) and gradually increase if needed.

CREATE YOUR OWN TINCTURE
TINCTURE NAME & SPECIFIC AILMENT OR CONCERN:

INGREDIENTS:

1. -
2. -
3. -
4. -
5. -

PREPARATION:

Combine equal parts of each herb (e.g., 1 ounce or 30 grams each) in a glass jar. Cover them with vodka or another high-proof alcohol, ensuring all the herbs are submerged. Seal the jar tightly.

Shake the jar daily for 4-6 weeks to allow the alcohol to extract the medicinal compounds.

STORAGE:

Store the jar in a cool, dark place. After 4-6 weeks, strain the tincture using cheesecloth or a fine-mesh strainer, and transfer the liquid into amber glass dropper bottles for easy use. This tincture can be stored for up to 5 years.

ADDITIONAL INFORMATION:

Remember to label your tinctures with the ingredients and date of preparation. Start with small doses (e.g., a dropperful) and gradually increase if needed.

CREATE YOUR OWN TINCTURE
TINCTURE NAME & SPECIFIC AILMENT OR CONCERN:

INGREDIENTS:
1. -
2. -
3. -
4. -
5. -

PREPARATION:

Combine equal parts of each herb (e.g., 1 ounce or 30 grams each) in a glass jar. Cover them with vodka or another high-proof alcohol, ensuring all the herbs are submerged. Seal the jar tightly.

Shake the jar daily for 4-6 weeks to allow the alcohol to extract the medicinal compounds.

STORAGE:

Store the jar in a cool, dark place. After 4-6 weeks, strain the tincture using cheesecloth or a fine-mesh strainer, and transfer the liquid into amber glass dropper bottles for easy use. This tincture can be stored for up to 5 years.

ADDITIONAL INFORMATION:

**Remember to label your tinctures with the ingredients and date of preparation. Start with small doses (e.g., a dropperful) and gradually increase if needed.**

TINCTURE NAME & SPECIFIC AILMENT OR CONCERN:

INGREDIENTS:

1. -
2. -
3. -
4. -
5. -

PREPARATION:

Combine equal parts of each herb (e.g., 1 ounce or 30 grams each) in a glass jar. Cover them with vodka or another high-proof alcohol, ensuring all the herbs are submerged. Seal the jar tightly.

Shake the jar daily for 4-6 weeks to allow the alcohol to extract the medicinal compounds.

STORAGE:

Store the jar in a cool, dark place. After 4-6 weeks, strain the tincture using cheesecloth or a fine-mesh strainer, and transfer the liquid into amber glass dropper bottles for easy use. This tincture can be stored for up to 5 years.

ADDITIONAL INFORMATION:

Remember to label your tinctures with the ingredients and date of preparation. Start with small doses (e.g., a dropperful) and gradually increase if needed.

TINCTURE NAME & SPECIFIC AILMENT OR CONCERN:

INGREDIENTS:

1. -
2. -
3. -
4. -
5. -

PREPARATION:

Combine equal parts of each herb (e.g., 1 ounce or 30 grams each) in a glass jar. Cover them with vodka or another high-proof alcohol, ensuring all the herbs are submerged. Seal the jar tightly.

Shake the jar daily for 4-6 weeks to allow the alcohol to extract the medicinal compounds.

STORAGE:

Store the jar in a cool, dark place. After 4-6 weeks, strain the tincture using cheesecloth or a fine-mesh strainer, and transfer the liquid into amber glass dropper bottles for easy use. This tincture can be stored for up to 5 years.

ADDITIONAL INFORMATION:

Remember to label your tinctures with the ingredients and date of preparation. Start with small doses (e.g., a dropperful) and gradually increase if needed.

CREATE YOUR OWN TINCTURE
TINCTURE NAME & SPECIFIC AILMENT OR CONCERN:

INGREDIENTS:
1. -
2. -
3. -
4. -
5. -

PREPARATION:

Combine equal parts of each herb (e.g., 1 ounce or 30 grams each) in a glass jar. Cover them with vodka or another high-proof alcohol, ensuring all the herbs are submerged. Seal the jar tightly.

Shake the jar daily for 4-6 weeks to allow the alcohol to extract the medicinal compounds.

STORAGE:

Store the jar in a cool, dark place. After 4-6 weeks, strain the tincture using cheesecloth or a fine-mesh strainer, and transfer the liquid into amber glass dropper bottles for easy use. This tincture can be stored for up to 5 years.

ADDITIONAL INFORMATION:

Remember to label your tinctures with the ingredients and date of preparation. Start with small doses (e.g., a dropperful) and gradually increase if needed.

CREATE YOUR OWN TINCTURE
TINCTURE NAME & SPECIFIC AILMENT OR CONCERN:

INGREDIENTS:

1. -
2. -
3. -
4. -
5. -

PREPARATION:

Combine equal parts of each herb (e.g., 1 ounce or 30 grams each) in a glass jar. Cover them with vodka or another high-proof alcohol, ensuring all the herbs are submerged. Seal the jar tightly.

Shake the jar daily for 4-6 weeks to allow the alcohol to extract the medicinal compounds.

STORAGE:

Store the jar in a cool, dark place. After 4-6 weeks, strain the tincture using cheesecloth or a fine-mesh strainer, and transfer the liquid into amber glass dropper bottles for easy use. This tincture can be stored for up to 5 years.

ADDITIONAL INFORMATION:

Remember to label your tinctures with the ingredients and date of preparation. Start with small doses (e.g., a dropperful) and gradually increase if needed.

CREATE YOUR OWN TINCTURE
TINCTURE NAME & SPECIFIC AILMENT OR CONCERN:

INGREDIENTS:

1. -
2. -
3. -
4. -
5. -

PREPARATION:

Combine equal parts of each herb (e.g., 1 ounce or 30 grams each) in a glass jar. Cover them with vodka or another high-proof alcohol, ensuring all the herbs are submerged. Seal the jar tightly.

Shake the jar daily for 4-6 weeks to allow the alcohol to extract the medicinal compounds.

STORAGE:

Store the jar in a cool, dark place. After 4-6 weeks, strain the tincture using cheesecloth or a fine-mesh strainer, and transfer the liquid into amber glass dropper bottles for easy use. This tincture can be stored for up to 5 years.

ADDITIONAL INFORMATION:

Remember to label your tinctures with the ingredients and date of preparation. Start with small doses (e.g., a dropperful) and gradually increase if needed.

CREATE YOUR OWN TINCTURE
TINCTURE NAME & SPECIFIC AILMENT OR CONCERN:

INGREDIENTS:
1. -
2. -
3. -
4. -
5. -

PREPARATION:
Combine equal parts of each herb (e.g., 1 ounce or 30 grams each) in a glass jar. Cover them with vodka or another high-proof alcohol, ensuring all the herbs are submerged. Seal the jar tightly.

Shake the jar daily for 4-6 weeks to allow the alcohol to extract the medicinal compounds.

STORAGE:
Store the jar in a cool, dark place. After 4-6 weeks, strain the tincture using cheesecloth or a fine-mesh strainer, and transfer the liquid into amber glass dropper bottles for easy use. This tincture can be stored for up to 5 years.

ADDITIONAL INFORMATION:

Remember to label your tinctures with the ingredients and date of preparation. Start with small doses (e.g., a dropperful) and gradually increase if needed.

CREATE YOUR OWN TINCTURE

TINCTURE NAME & SPECIFIC AILMENT OR CONCERN:

INGREDIENTS:

1. -
2. -
3. -
4. -
5. -

PREPARATION:

Combine equal parts of each herb (e.g., 1 ounce or 30 grams each) in a glass jar. Cover them with vodka or another high-proof alcohol, ensuring all the herbs are submerged. Seal the jar tightly.

Shake the jar daily for 4-6 weeks to allow the alcohol to extract the medicinal compounds.

STORAGE:

Store the jar in a cool, dark place. After 4-6 weeks, strain the tincture using cheesecloth or a fine-mesh strainer, and transfer the liquid into amber glass dropper bottles for easy use. This tincture can be stored for up to 5 years.

ADDITIONAL INFORMATION:

**Remember to label your tinctures with the ingredients and date of preparation. Start with small doses (e.g., a dropperful) and gradually increase if needed.**

TINCTURE NAME & SPECIFIC AILMENT OR CONCERN:

INGREDIENTS:

1. -
2. -
3. -
4. -
5. -

PREPARATION:

Combine equal parts of each herb (e.g., 1 ounce or 30 grams each) in a glass jar. Cover them with vodka or another high-proof alcohol, ensuring all the herbs are submerged. Seal the jar tightly.

Shake the jar daily for 4-6 weeks to allow the alcohol to extract the medicinal compounds.

STORAGE:

Store the jar in a cool, dark place. After 4-6 weeks, strain the tincture using cheesecloth or a fine-mesh strainer, and transfer the liquid into amber glass dropper bottles for easy use. This tincture can be stored for up to 5 years.

ADDITIONAL INFORMATION:

Remember to label your tinctures with the ingredients and date of preparation. Start with small doses (e.g., a dropperful) and gradually increase if needed.

CREATE YOUR OWN TINCTURE
TINCTURE NAME & SPECIFIC AILMENT OR CONCERN:

INGREDIENTS:

1. -
2. -
3. -
4. -
5. -

PREPARATION:

Combine equal parts of each herb (e.g., 1 ounce or 30 grams each) in a glass jar. Cover them with vodka or another high-proof alcohol, ensuring all the herbs are submerged. Seal the jar tightly.

Shake the jar daily for 4-6 weeks to allow the alcohol to extract the medicinal compounds.

STORAGE:

Store the jar in a cool, dark place. After 4-6 weeks, strain the tincture using cheesecloth or a fine-mesh strainer, and transfer the liquid into amber glass dropper bottles for easy use. This tincture can be stored for up to 5 years.

ADDITIONAL INFORMATION:

**Remember to label your tinctures with the ingredients and date of preparation. Start with small doses (e.g., a dropperful) and gradually increase if needed.**

CREATE YOUR OWN TINCTURE
TINCTURE NAME & SPECIFIC AILMENT OR CONCERN:

INGREDIENTS:

1. -
2. -
3. -
4. -
5. -

PREPARATION:

Combine equal parts of each herb (e.g., 1 ounce or 30 grams each) in a glass jar. Cover them with vodka or another high-proof alcohol, ensuring all the herbs are submerged. Seal the jar tightly.

Shake the jar daily for 4-6 weeks to allow the alcohol to extract the medicinal compounds.

STORAGE:

Store the jar in a cool, dark place. After 4-6 weeks, strain the tincture using cheesecloth or a fine-mesh strainer, and transfer the liquid into amber glass dropper bottles for easy use. This tincture can be stored for up to 5 years.

ADDITIONAL INFORMATION:

Remember to label your tinctures with the ingredients and date of preparation. Start with small doses (e.g., a dropperful) and gradually increase if needed.

CREATE YOUR OWN TINCTURE
TINCTURE NAME & SPECIFIC AILMENT OR CONCERN:

INGREDIENTS:

1. -
2. -
3. -
4. -
5. -

PREPARATION:

Combine equal parts of each herb (e.g., 1 ounce or 30 grams each) in a glass jar. Cover them with vodka or another high-proof alcohol, ensuring all the herbs are submerged. Seal the jar tightly.

Shake the jar daily for 4-6 weeks to allow the alcohol to extract the medicinal compounds.

STORAGE:

Store the jar in a cool, dark place. After 4-6 weeks, strain the tincture using cheesecloth or a fine-mesh strainer, and transfer the liquid into amber glass dropper bottles for easy use. This tincture can be stored for up to 5 years.

ADDITIONAL INFORMATION:

**Remember to label your tinctures with the ingredients and date of preparation. Start with small doses (e.g., a dropperful) and gradually increase if needed.**

CREATE YOUR OWN TINCTURE
TINCTURE NAME & SPECIFIC AILMENT OR CONCERN:

INGREDIENTS:
1. -
2. -
3. -
4. -
5. -

PREPARATION:

Combine equal parts of each herb (e.g., 1 ounce or 30 grams each) in a glass jar. Cover them with vodka or another high-proof alcohol, ensuring all the herbs are submerged. Seal the jar tightly.

Shake the jar daily for 4-6 weeks to allow the alcohol to extract the medicinal compounds.

STORAGE:

Store the jar in a cool, dark place. After 4-6 weeks, strain the tincture using cheesecloth or a fine-mesh strainer, and transfer the liquid into amber glass dropper bottles for easy use. This tincture can be stored for up to 5 years.

ADDITIONAL INFORMATION:

Remember to label your tinctures with the ingredients and date of preparation. Start with small doses (e.g., a dropperful) and gradually increase if needed.

CREATE YOUR OWN TINCTURE
TINCTURE NAME & SPECIFIC AILMENT OR CONCERN:

INGREDIENTS:

1. -
2. -
3. -
4. -
5. -

PREPARATION:

Combine equal parts of each herb (e.g., 1 ounce or 30 grams each) in a glass jar. Cover them with vodka or another high-proof alcohol, ensuring all the herbs are submerged. Seal the jar tightly.

Shake the jar daily for 4-6 weeks to allow the alcohol to extract the medicinal compounds.

STORAGE:

Store the jar in a cool, dark place. After 4-6 weeks, strain the tincture using cheesecloth or a fine-mesh strainer, and transfer the liquid into amber glass dropper bottles for easy use. This tincture can be stored for up to 5 years.

ADDITIONAL INFORMATION:

**Remember to label your tinctures with the ingredients and date of preparation. Start with small doses (e.g., a dropperful) and gradually increase if needed.**

CREATE YOUR OWN TINCTURE
TINCTURE NAME & SPECIFIC AILMENT OR CONCERN:

INGREDIENTS:

1. -
2. -
3. -
4. -
5. -

PREPARATION:

Combine equal parts of each herb (e.g., 1 ounce or 30 grams each) in a glass jar. Cover them with vodka or another high-proof alcohol, ensuring all the herbs are submerged. Seal the jar tightly.

Shake the jar daily for 4-6 weeks to allow the alcohol to extract the medicinal compounds.

STORAGE:

Store the jar in a cool, dark place. After 4-6 weeks, strain the tincture using cheesecloth or a fine-mesh strainer, and transfer the liquid into amber glass dropper bottles for easy use. This tincture can be stored for up to 5 years.

ADDITIONAL INFORMATION:

Remember to label your tinctures with the ingredients and date of preparation. Start with small doses (e.g., a dropperful) and gradually increase if needed.

CREATE YOUR OWN TINCTURE
TINCTURE NAME & SPECIFIC AILMENT OR CONCERN:

INGREDIENTS:

1. -
2. -
3. -
4. -
5. -

PREPARATION:

Combine equal parts of each herb (e.g., 1 ounce or 30 grams each) in a glass jar. Cover them with vodka or another high-proof alcohol, ensuring all the herbs are submerged. Seal the jar tightly.

Shake the jar daily for 4-6 weeks to allow the alcohol to extract the medicinal compounds.

STORAGE:

Store the jar in a cool, dark place. After 4-6 weeks, strain the tincture using cheesecloth or a fine-mesh strainer, and transfer the liquid into amber glass dropper bottles for easy use. This tincture can be stored for up to 5 years.

ADDITIONAL INFORMATION:

Remember to label your tinctures with the ingredients and date of preparation. Start with small doses (e.g., a dropperful) and gradually increase if needed.

CREATE YOUR OWN TINCTURE
TINCTURE NAME & SPECIFIC AILMENT OR CONCERN:

INGREDIENTS:

1. -
2. -
3. -
4. -
5. -

PREPARATION:

Combine equal parts of each herb (e.g., 1 ounce or 30 grams each) in a glass jar. Cover them with vodka or another high-proof alcohol, ensuring all the herbs are submerged. Seal the jar tightly.

Shake the jar daily for 4-6 weeks to allow the alcohol to extract the medicinal compounds.

STORAGE:

Store the jar in a cool, dark place. After 4-6 weeks, strain the tincture using cheesecloth or a fine-mesh strainer, and transfer the liquid into amber glass dropper bottles for easy use. This tincture can be stored for up to 5 years.

ADDITIONAL INFORMATION:

**Remember to label your tinctures with the ingredients and date of preparation. Start with small doses (e.g., a dropperful) and gradually increase if needed.**

CREATE YOUR OWN TINCTURE
TINCTURE NAME & SPECIFIC AILMENT OR CONCERN:

INGREDIENTS:

1. -
2. -
3. -
4. -
5. -

PREPARATION:

Combine equal parts of each herb (e.g., 1 ounce or 30 grams each) in a glass jar. Cover them with vodka or another high-proof alcohol, ensuring all the herbs are submerged. Seal the jar tightly.

Shake the jar daily for 4-6 weeks to allow the alcohol to extract the medicinal compounds.

STORAGE:

Store the jar in a cool, dark place. After 4-6 weeks, strain the tincture using cheesecloth or a fine-mesh strainer, and transfer the liquid into amber glass dropper bottles for easy use. This tincture can be stored for up to 5 years.

ADDITIONAL INFORMATION:

Remember to label your tinctures with the ingredients and date of preparation. Start with small doses (e.g., a dropperful) and gradually increase if needed.

CREATE YOUR OWN TINCTURE
TINCTURE NAME & SPECIFIC AILMENT OR CONCERN:

INGREDIENTS:

1. -
2. -
3. -
4. -
5. -

PREPARATION:

Combine equal parts of each herb (e.g., 1 ounce or 30 grams each) in a glass jar. Cover them with vodka or another high-proof alcohol, ensuring all the herbs are submerged. Seal the jar tightly.

Shake the jar daily for 4-6 weeks to allow the alcohol to extract the medicinal compounds.

STORAGE:

Store the jar in a cool, dark place. After 4-6 weeks, strain the tincture using cheesecloth or a fine-mesh strainer, and transfer the liquid into amber glass dropper bottles for easy use. This tincture can be stored for up to 5 years.

ADDITIONAL INFORMATION:

Remember to label your tinctures with the ingredients and date of preparation. Start with small doses (e.g., a dropperful) and gradually increase if needed.

INGREDIENTS:

1. -
2. -
3. -
4. -
5. -

PREPARATION:

Combine equal parts of each herb (e.g., 1 ounce or 30 grams each) in a glass jar. Cover them with vodka or another high-proof alcohol, ensuring all the herbs are submerged. Seal the jar tightly.

Shake the jar daily for 4-6 weeks to allow the alcohol to extract the medicinal compounds.

STORAGE:

Store the jar in a cool, dark place. After 4-6 weeks, strain the tincture using cheesecloth or a fine-mesh strainer, and transfer the liquid into amber glass dropper bottles for easy use. This tincture can be stored for up to 5 years.

ADDITIONAL INFORMATION:

**Remember to label your tinctures with the ingredients and date of preparation. Start with small doses (e.g., a dropperful) and gradually increase if needed**

CREATE YOUR OWN TINCTURE
TINCTURE NAME & SPECIFIC AILMENT OR CONCERN:

INGREDIENTS:

1. -
2. -
3. -
4. -
5. -

PREPARATION:

Combine equal parts of each herb (e.g., 1 ounce or 30 grams each) in a glass jar. Cover them with vodka or another high-proof alcohol, ensuring all the herbs are submerged. Seal the jar tightly.

Shake the jar daily for 4-6 weeks to allow the alcohol to extract the medicinal compounds.

STORAGE:

Store the jar in a cool, dark place. After 4-6 weeks, strain the tincture using cheesecloth or a fine-mesh strainer, and transfer the liquid into amber glass dropper bottles for easy use. This tincture can be stored for up to 5 years.

ADDITIONAL INFORMATION:

Remember to label your tinctures with the ingredients and date of preparation. Start with small doses (e.g., a dropperful) and gradually increase if needed.

www.ingramcontent.com/pod-product-compliance
Lightning Source LLC
Chambersburg PA
CBHW051258250726
48656CB00004B/1365